Hairy Stories

HAIRY STORIES

Photographs by Beate Brosche, texts by Gudrun Patricia Pott

EDITION STEMMLE

Contents

Foreword
7

Hairy Stories
Interesting, amusing and totally incredible stories from the history and culture of hair.
A text full of laughs and surprises
9

Figaro in his Prime
Hairstyles from the modest to the outlandish
21

Hairy Times
Profiles of hairstyles
77

Frank Schäfer
Germany's most daring hairstylist
79

Horst Chudy/Markus Krause
Hair-tours – a hair-raising trip through Berlin staged by
two very unusual hair artists
87

Andreas Hintz
Unique wigs by the "Atelier Perrückt" in Hamburg
107

Hairy – Hairier – Hairiest
Permanent lab, witch's blood and tickly curls –
Photo-impressions of heads and hair
113

Foreword

There are innumerable "hairy stories," in the literal and in the figurative sense. A number of them have been collected in this book in words and pictures. Preceding all of these, however, we would like to tell a personal, hair-raising story with a conciliatory end, namely this book. It goes like this:

A little girl accompanied her grandmother to the hairdresser's. It was time for a new permanent. Soon, grandmother was sitting under the hair-dryer, totally absorbed in her precious reading: all at home with the European royalty; all seemed well in the world. Everything about her was forgotten. Meanwhile, her granddaughter's split ends needed a trim. She was getting ready for her first day at school.

And disaster took its course: the hairdresser, "mean and nasty," got the appointments mixed up, grabbed her scissors and gave the scared child a radical short haircut with shaved nape and sideburns. Before the girl could protest, her long, blond hair was lying on the floor. The girl, far too timid, just let everything happen to her. Small, miserable, and petrified, she sat in the huge hairdresser's chair, hands cramped under the cape, much too large for her, fighting back her tears. The grandmother, now donning her new silver locks, hardly recognized her granddaughter. Oh, my goodness. But, what was gone, was gone. The child hated adults, gathered her cut-off hair from the floor, and took it home to store it away in a cigar box. Not until she was outside the salon, did she begin to cry and vowed never again to go to the hairdresser's.

24 years later, the girl had become photographer, Beate Brosche, she received a phone call from *STERN* magazine. Whether she had time to photograph a story. Sure! Without, at first, inquiring about the subject, Beate said yes. HAIRDRESSERS! That's just what she needed! In a meeting with editor Gudrun Pott, the photographer confessed her phobia. Now she just had to face it: daily visits to three or four scenes of horror, approaching her childhood enemy, armed with a camera. The team had a lot of fun meeting all kinds of different people. And, in the end, even Beate came to the conclusion: Hairdressers are nice people.

So much for the hair-raising story behind "Hairy Stories."

The Art Director's Club of Germany awarded us a prize for our work together. Yet, our subject "hair" did not let go of us. Further photo assignments followed. And, one day, we decided to take all our photo and text material and put together a book.

Beate Brosche and Gudrun Patricia Pott

Hairy Stories

A face too long, prominent ears, a flat back of the head, lax skin, thinning or graying hair and dandruff: mainly, beauty flaws of the fairer sex, often concealed in vain. Yet, there is one to whom everything is unveiled mercilessly: the hairdresser. To call him a mere craftsman, this Master of the Scissors? Much too common place! He is, much more, a magician, a consoler, a rescuer in dire need. This is because people always want to have exactly what has not been given unto them. This makes for quite a handsome living for the guild. As mediator between reality and wishful thinking, it is up to the Figaro of Hope to achieve that which nature has so steadfastly withheld.

Nobody but a plastic surgeon can alter a person's appearance as much as a hairdresser. That is why many consider him their confidant, as indispensable as their physician. They submit to his diagnosis, full of hope. After all, with the proper hair-do, a different color, quite a few things can be covered up. Washing, curling, drying: between cut, permanent, and hair-dryer, life takes on a whole new look.

For this dream, women readily offered hairdressers their heads, eight times annually (1996 statistics), doled out, on average, DM 54.60 ($30.30). The gentlemen went to the hairdresser's just as often but came away DM 30 ($ 16.60) cheaper. From the hairdresser way down in some Bavarian village, all the way up to Berlin's zany, fashionable scene, some 224,000 employees in 51,500 hairdresser shops in Germany offer complete service to their customers. Usually, not only hair service. At a good Figaro's, the customer is also brought into shape.

Grow as they will: that was alright for the 100,000 hairs on the head of a Neandertal. The celt had just been invented, when combs and barrettes were first being marketed. Our ancestors began styling themselves.

Hair has always been something of a mystery, at times even an enigma. It was a symbol of power, beauty, and youth, represented glory or defeat. The ancient Greek thinkers considered flowing hair and beards symbols of wisdom and kindness. The wives of Roman senators thought wigs of Germanic blond hair quite fashionable. Thank goodness, the days had passed, when shaved heads were considered a Teutonic sign of submission, and your honor was lost when your beard was cut off. Greek boys offered Apollo, the God of poetry and prophecy, their locks. The Philistine Delilah stole the Hebrew Samson's hair, thereby robbing him of all his power.

Today's sacrifices are to beauty and image. Show me your head and I will tell you who you are. For the German poet Goethe, it was "undeniable ... that hair color meant a difference in character." A popular saying, which particularly applies to females, goes: black devil, red witch, blond angel.

Nature has figured out quite cleverly where hair is supposed to grow. Always in search of hairy individuality, hairdressers have taken these spots in hand. Not only are eyebrows plucked and eyelashes dyed. Long is made short but with a "hair extension" the opposite can also come true. If you bring along much patience and DM 800 ($ 444.40), the pro will also conjure up the ever so desired lion's mane onto a stubbly head: all with braided and waxed genuine strands of hair. The perfect illusion for three months, after all. In Berlin's fashionable salons, even the intimate mop of hair (some also call it "battle hair") is not safe from Figaro. As a birthday surprise for one's sweetheart or as the crowning event for a tête-à-tête: a pubic hair-do, shaved into a design or given a shrill color. And, noble punks, in quest of the ultimate kick, have come upon "piercing," the latest rage. Nipples, navels, and vulvas are painfully drilled through, to be embellished with gold and silver hunks.

Once before, in the Middle Ages, the craft was bloody. Barber surgeons, predecessors of today's hairdressers, devoted themselves to the so-called "lower medicine." They performed tasks which privileged physicians considered in bad taste. With horrid instruments they pulled teeth, cupped, bled, treated abscesses, and performed amputations. A wooden hammer served as anesthesia. In 1610, the Wittenberger hairdresser, Jeremias Trautmann, even dared to perform a Cesarean section. The operation was partially successful: the boy lived, the mother died four weeks later. Sterilization was not yet under control.

During the days of Absolution, barbers turned toward modern artistry. They became wig-makers whose bizarre creations flowed down to the waist. These symbols of aristocratic decadence influenced Baroque and Rococo fashions. Naturalness was considered vulgar. Built-in flee traps were the only concession to nature.

In 1656, forty eight "perruquiers" made the Allonge wig mandatory at the court of Louis XIV. This caused the clergy some embarrassment as admission to the priesthood required a portion of the head to be shaven. This "tonsure" was somewhat of an open-line to the Lord. So, the hairdressers turned around and built the holy men a flap into their artificial splendor, which could be opened during services. Thus, they were able to satisfy both Holy Spirit and etiquette.

Acrobatics was the name of the women's game. The dizzy heights of the "Fontage-Towers", named after the duchess of the same name. The invention of the Sun King's mistress drove the Figaros to assemble their hair-dos standing on ladders. The face became the center of this hair-phenomenon. Owing to circumstances, madame preferred to sleep in an armchair.

All of Europe imitated this French craze. Business was booming. Saxony's secretary of state, Heinrich Graf von Brühl, was said to own 1,500 hair-pieces. This moved Frederick the Great to comment: "So many wigs for a man without a head." To boost the treasury, the princes collected taxes for the artificial splendor. So-called "wig-noses" went about ripping off false hair from unsuspecting wearers of artificial mops of hair. This method of verifying the mandatory tax seal often lead to brawls.

The period before the 1848 Revolution threw hairdressers into a hefty crisis. Powdered artificialness was out.

To the stubborn, young men of the German Students' Association, long, naturally flowing hair or combed across the forehead, and sideburns were symbols of progressive political conviction. This aroused the government's suspicions. 120 years later, Flower-Power hippies once again intimidated the Establishment with their long mops, and upset good, civil families with arguments between fathers and sons, and drove the guild of hairdressers into sheer desperation with their cry: "Let it live, your hair."

Despite this fleeting, mainly, male refusal, the hairy business gained an ever-increasing circle of female customers, who proved to be particularly willing to suffer. Many a head was scorched, using the permanent apparatus invented by Ludwig Nessler in 1906. The temperature of this horrid monstrosity could reach 120 °C (360 °F). Meanwhile, three kilos (6.5 lbs) of metal curlers tore away at the esteemed customer's head.

The gentlemen, less endowed with patience in matters of beauty, were again given conventional hair-cuts and relaxing shaves. They bought their fancy "rubber wares" discretely from Figaro and were grateful purchasers of all mixtures that promised them the one and only: a full head of hair. Despite grandmother's traditional prescriptions and innumerable, and at times, devilish tinctures and medical fertilizers, the results remained questionable. Up until this day, hairdressers and physicians are at a loss as to growth and disappearance on the shiny, pergament-like fallow of the male head.

The male's mark of Cain drives the defeated to questionable treatments again and again: anything to save at least the last few hairs or, if worst comes to worst, to conjure up a bit of fluff. Electrical 12-volt-fields are supposed to expedite growth, classical music is said to stimulate hair roots, meditation is implored, as a last resort, as power to the spirit. Or you court the knife. Hundreds, even thousands of tiny pieces of skin from the head, with one to four own hairs, are transplanted into tiny prepared holes onto the bald spots. Here, too, the long-lasting success remains to be seen: existing hair has merely been spread out sparingly. Nonetheless, each year some 7,000 men subject themselves to this costly procedure. Not seldom, 800–1,000 transplantations are necessary. Very quickly, that can add up to DM 10,000–15,000 ($ 5,555–$ 8,333).

There are many reasons for hair loss: improper diet, infections, fever, hormone problems. But for 95% of all men, baldness is inherited. It does them no good that every healthy hair, after four to six years of growth, takes a break or says goodbye forever. A thick bulb of horn cells affixes it to the skin. When growth ceases, the anker loosens after three to six months, the hair falls out, a new one grows back, or doesn't. The average loss of 100 hairs per day is normal. But for "alopecina androgenetica", plain old baldness, an incalculable fate for a third of all men, there is no cure.

Hairdressers profess the toupee as the rescue. Most times, it is a bit too thick or pulled down too far over the forehead, so as not to arouse suspicion. There are supposed to be some 80,000 who wear toupees in Germany. There are no concrete numbers. The knotted replacement is taboo. Whoever wears it, keeps the secret to himself. Not like in Japan, where it is considered unmannerly not to cover one's bald head with a second head of hair, the German dies of embarrassment: covering up long-gone hair with false volume is deceitful. This is why producers and sales people are also particularly discreet with intimate orders for pubic hair toupees. They care about their anxious customers' image.

The vain and bald construction tycoon, Jürgen Schneider, responsible for the biggest real estate bankruptcy in the Federal Republic of Germany, went to his Figaro every three weeks for a back hair trim and to have his hair pieces fluffed up with water vapor, as his hairdresser, Gerd Köpkes, revealed to the yellow press after bankruptcy. Every two years, Schneider bought a new toupee for DM 2,000 ($ 1,110).

If, last century, vanishing hair was considered the bill for leading a dissolute life, then every contemporary fellow-sufferer should gather fresh hope (woman have been admiring the likes of Yul Brunner and Telly Savallas for some time) and simply accept alleged special sexual powers as the consolation all bald men deserve.

From a legal point of view, the guild of hairdressers faces a delicate issue. Hair is considered a part of the body. By cutting or clipping it, the hairdresser is committing (permissable) bodily harm. Seldom, though, does this lead to as radical a protest as in the case of a 22-year-old Dutchman. His hairdresser, instead of giving him a trim, chopped off 30 centimeters (12 inches), whereupon the Dutchman smashed his salon to pieces.

The belief in the power of hair is substantial. In the fairy-tale world, Rapunzel lets down twenty yards of her golden mane out of her prison tower to allow her fairy-tale prince to climb up to her. And the son of poor people gains the king's daughter as his wife when he presents the devil's greedy father-in-law three of her golden hairs.

In the magical world of Sandra, who calls herself a witch, hair means everything. In Munich, where she runs Germany's only witch shop, she knows how to cure broken hearts and infidelity with the hairs of her customers' partners. In various rites, they are burned, affixed to dolls or tied together with those of the lovesick customer. All with the aim that this magic will return the lost love.

Witch Sandra believes in hair-power so much that she would never leave one behind in her hair brush. Far too great is her fear that someone might harm or gain power over her. And, she only gets a hair trim once a year. Of course, not by a hairdresser, but by a girlfriend, who is a witch herself.

The red-maned hairdresser, Ute Jacobs, from Berlin swears by the magical power of the full moon. On such nights, she organizes occult haircutting sessions with oracles and love potions. Her colleague, Jonny Pazzo, who was German pop singer Nena's inspiration, not only celebrates hairiness in his Berlin "in"-studio but also puts the power of crystals to work. Pazzo really believes that amethyst, the stone of belief, wards off seduction, magic, and purifies his customers' souls.

Other experts rely on the laws of chemistry to tackle such problems as greasy hair or hair that is too dry, brittle or dull. They promise their customers more self-confidence with a vast palette of hair-care products. For this promise, customers are willing to pay a lot. Each year, Germans spend 4.6 billion DM ($ 2.5 billion). Rewarding for an industry that manufactures 150,000 tons of hair-care products annually for the German market. Despite the general recession, its numbers are ever increasing. The constant new presentation of different products costs this line of business enormous sums.

The French company L'Oréal invested 480 million DM ($ 220 Million). Their annual turnover of 18 billion DM ($ 10 billion) worldwide made them Number One in the hair-care market and their round-the-clock research development.

It is a lengthy process before a new product is ready for the market. Seventy chemists at the research center in Clichy require 80,000 strands of hair to test the durability of a single hair color. The colored hairtufts, each weighing precisely one gram (0.04 oz), are washed, shaken, sprayed, and stretched again and again. Finally, these fruits of research are tested on live objects. Every day, some 600 mostly female test persons in 206 seats have their hair washed, curled, and colored. Conscientiously, the company's hairdressers record all observations and findings about the new product as they run through their final check.

The Figaros are also quite engaged in meeting their clientele's needs. And those needs vary as much as the atmosphere of the different salons. There are those, who have aged with their customers in their slightly dusty, cozy living rooms. There's coffee from a thermos and dramatic reading stuff about Europe's royalty. A great gossip-meet for all the news not in the papers. An empathetic hairdresser listens to private secrets and sorrows, which nobody at home cares to hear. They know each other and appreciate this familiarity. Anthing new arouses suspicion. Only the head is restored. And often, three ladies, whose ages together add up to 240, sit in a row, having their hair permed, the good old way.

How different, the beauty temple, embellished in chrome and steel, where the boss calls himself hair-stylist, the image-designer, who works under continually throbbing music. The appointment book is filled up, and the Master of the Scissors fumbles around on three heads simultaneously. Sometimes, the service offered is quite unique: a hairdresser in Düsseldorf, located in the stylish Kö-Gallery, attracts customers with an "oxygen-oasis," where the stress-plagued may inhale under a mask to recover their breath. In a New York salon, a fortune-teller, a dream analyst, and an astrologer help pass the waiting time. And in Australian Adelaide, in the early nineties, a topless barber parlor was the big hit. Despite its prices, that were twice as high, it outdid the competition.

The guild has long become presentable. Being familiar with the hair-artist is considered quite chic within kissy-kissy circles. Gloria, the formerly wild Princess of Thurn and Taxis, helped hers get his career started. Her Highness thanked Gerhard Meir from Munich for his PR success in creating her wild hair-dos by writing him: "Honey, honey, what have you made of me," and ever so devoted, "Magician, I'm all yours."

Figaro in his Prime

From the early barber down in Bavaria all the way up to the noble coiffeur in Hamburg, from the bizarre-punky hair-artist in Berlin to the traditional hairdresser in Meissen, where everything has remained as it was in old East Germany: a journey through German hairdressers' salons, from bourgeois to wild.

ALL COMBED and spruced up: childhood memories relived. Chopped hair was a symbol of parental power; a visit to the hairdresser's often turned into a nightmare. Davide also is skeptical as Walter Löwenberg gives him a traditional cut. Quite practical: the master lives right behind his salon from the 60's at the Hamburg Port. His wife runs a little fast-food place across the street, where customers can go for snack afterwards.

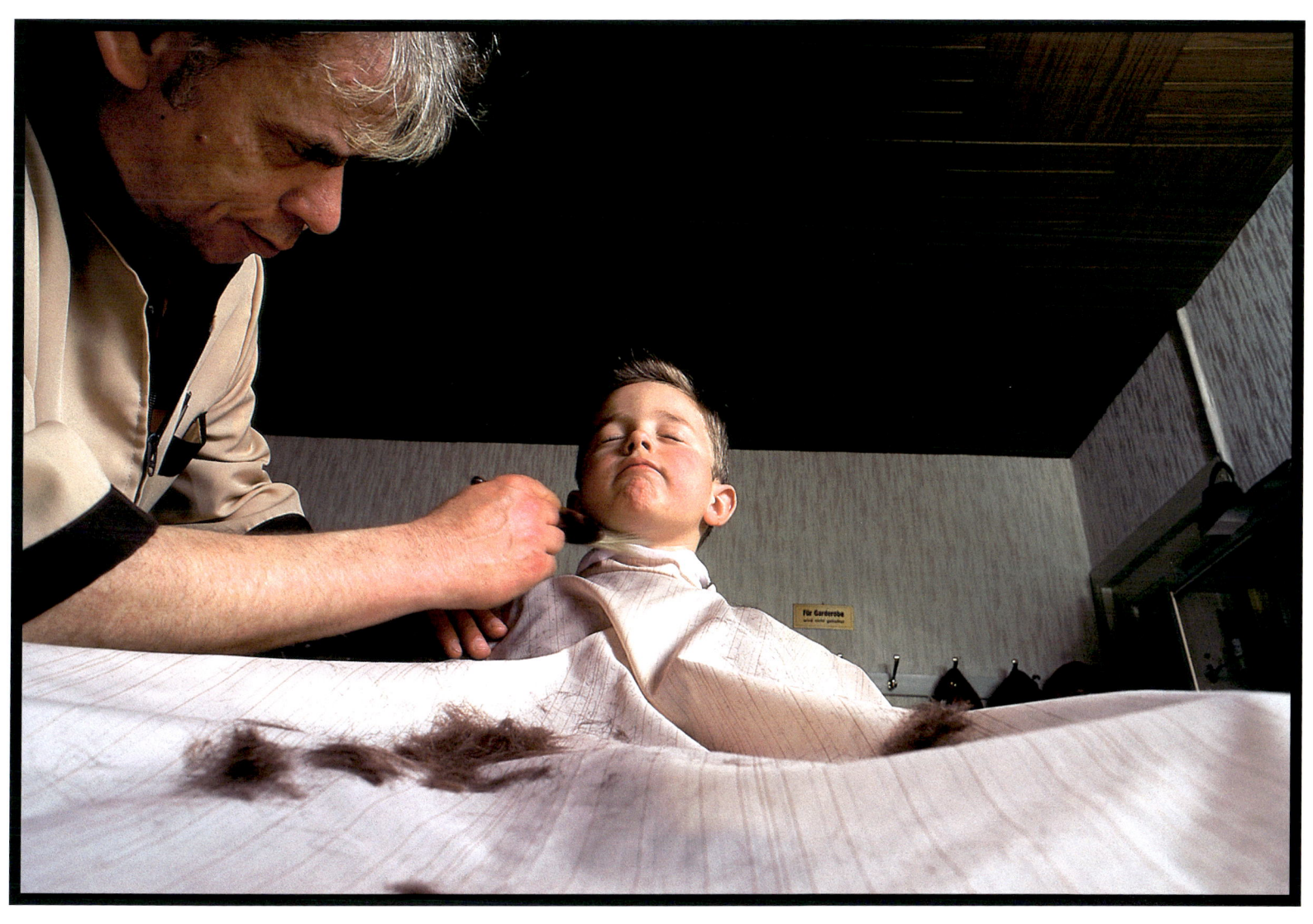

Walter Löwenberg/Hamburg

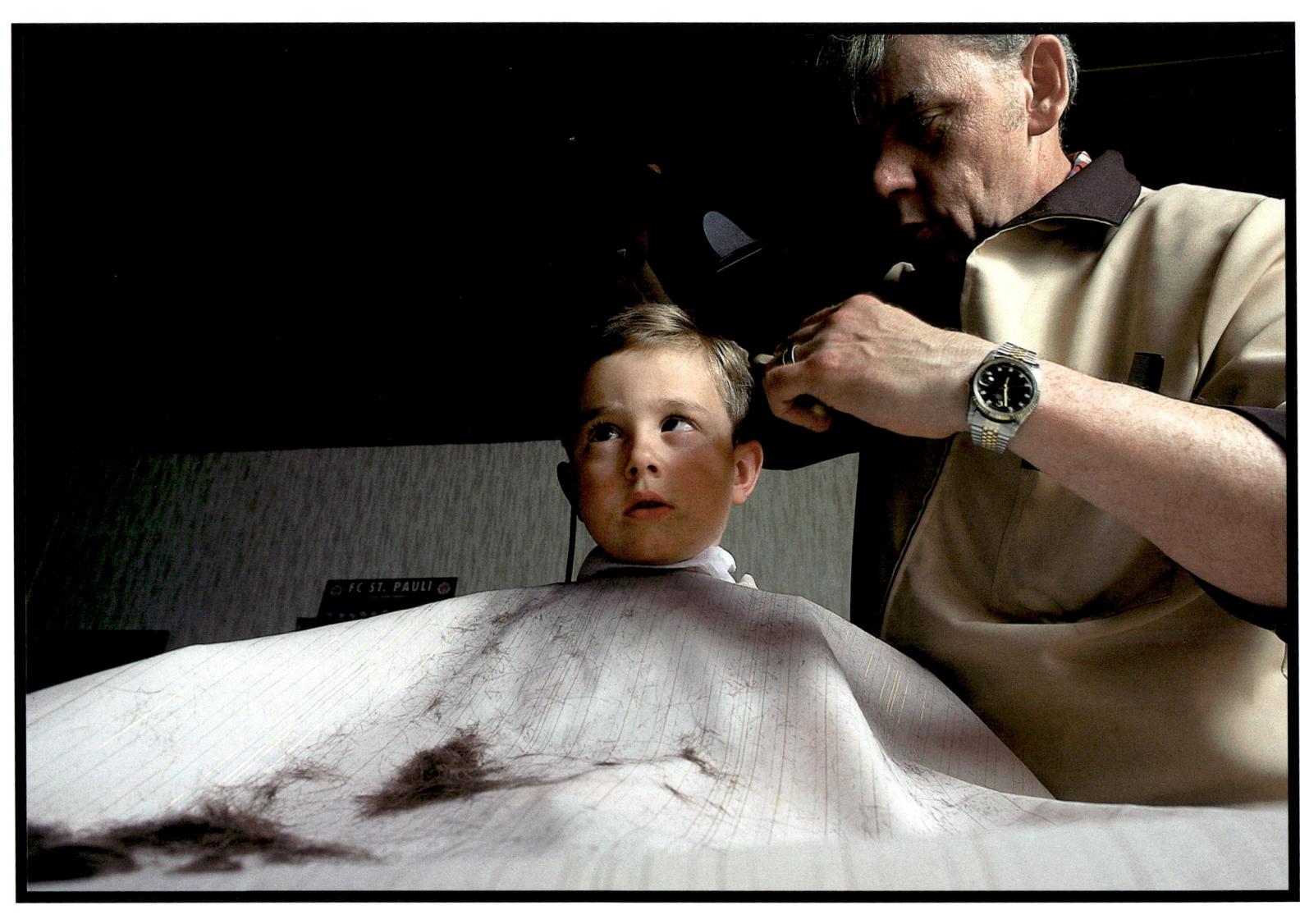

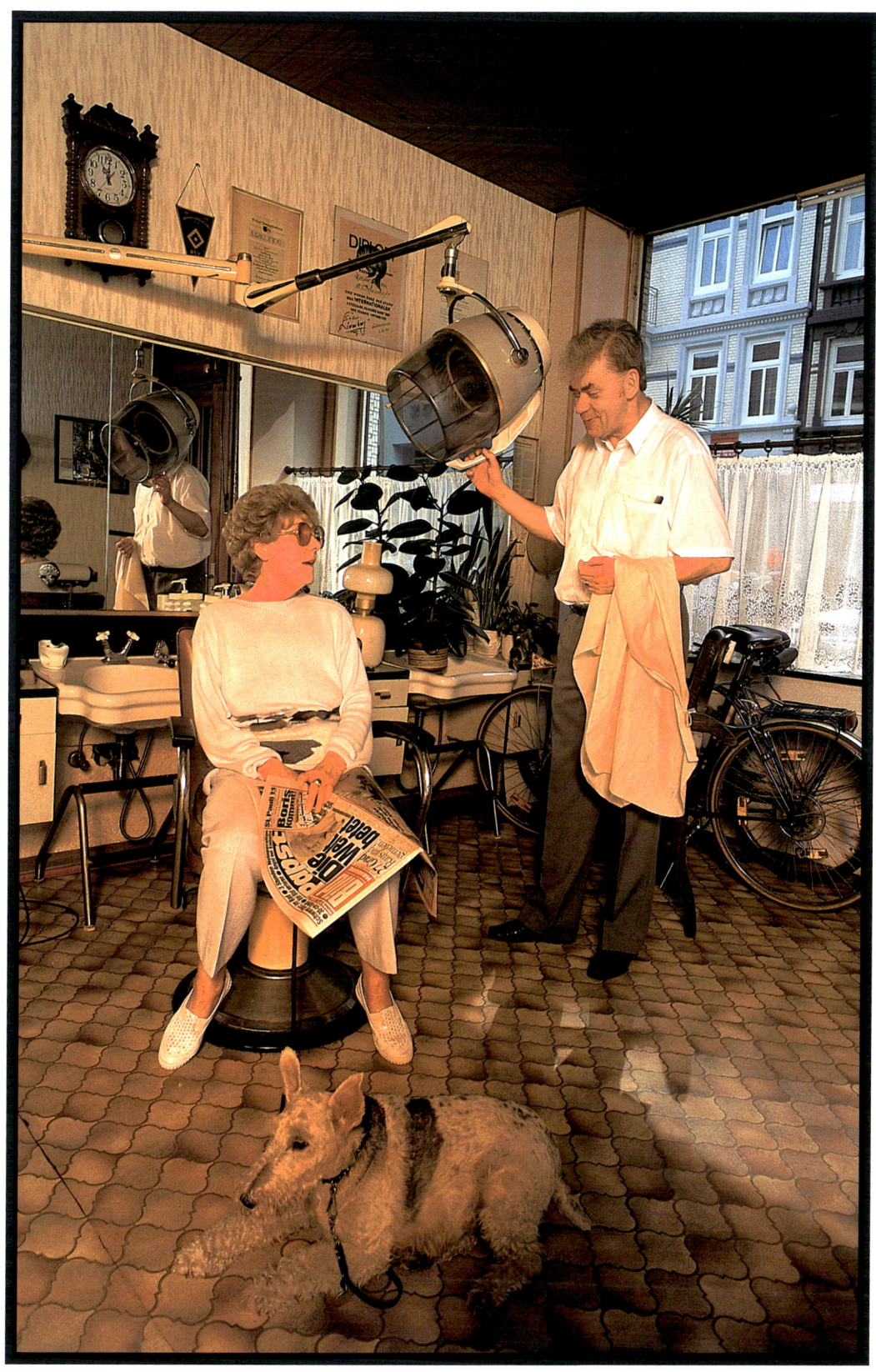

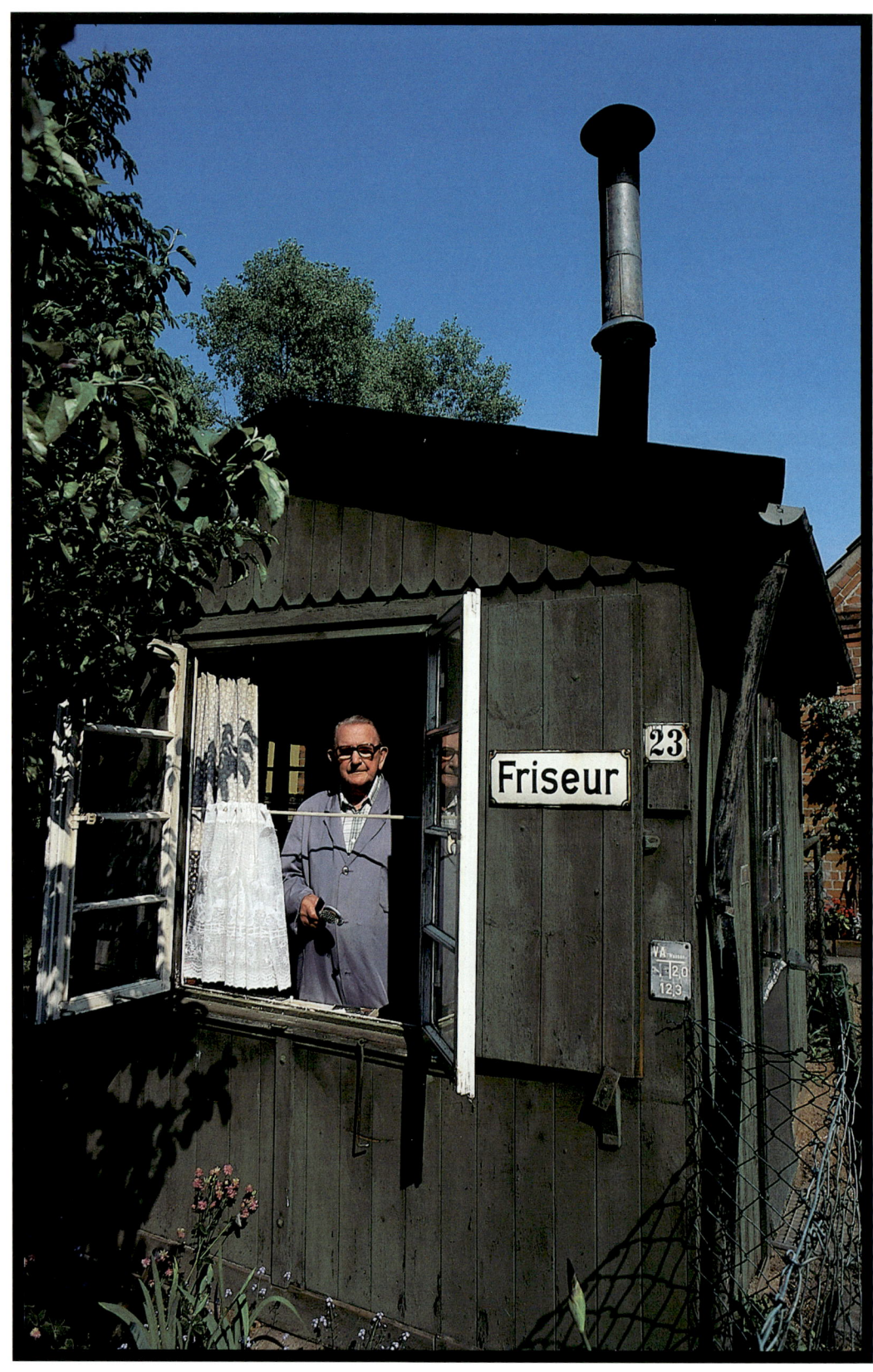

Herbert Benthien/Lübeck

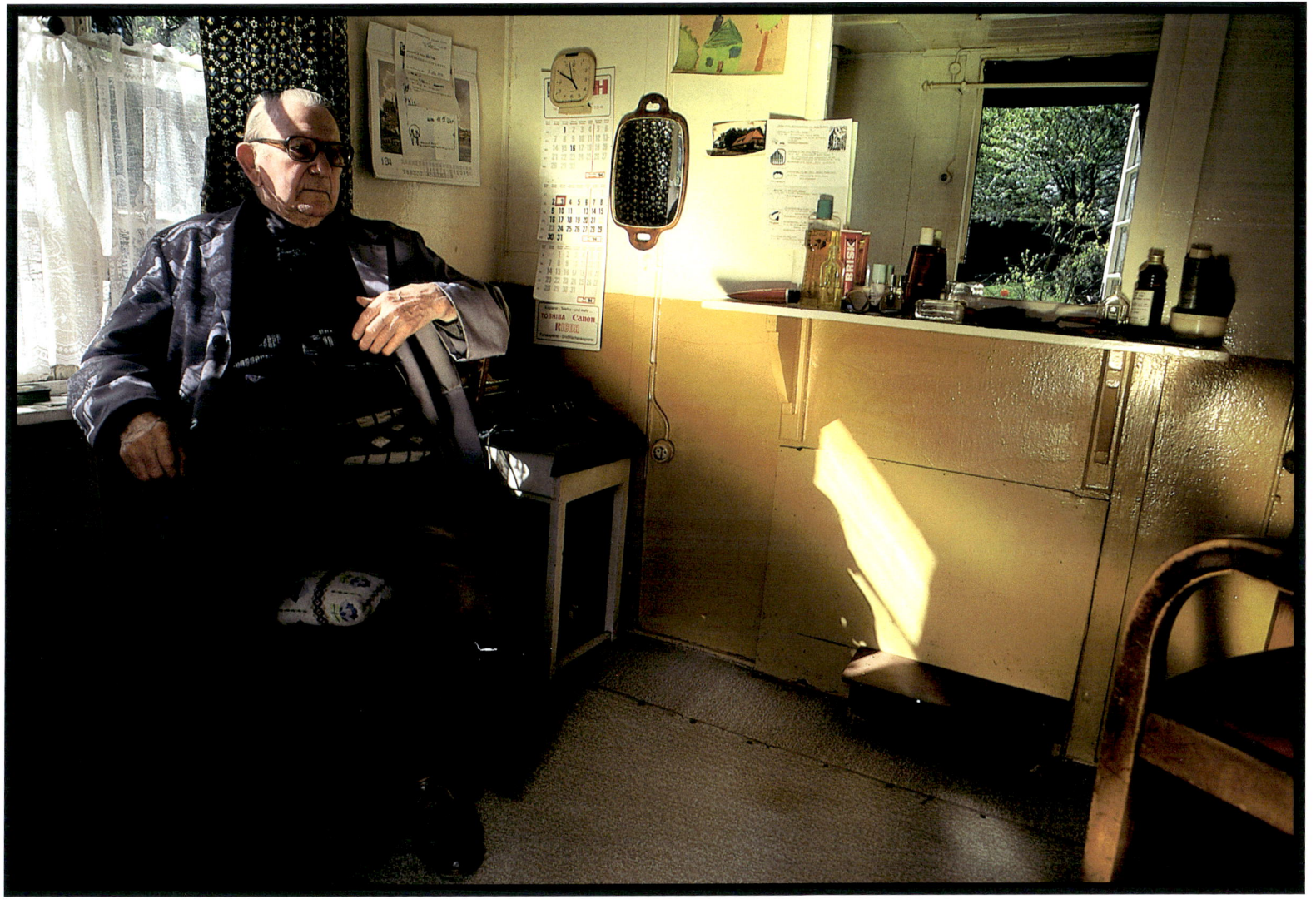

DESPITE HIS 95 YEARS, Germany's oldest hairdresser permits his scissors no rest. In 1916, Herbert Benthien became his uncle's apprentice for a weekly salary of 50 Pfennigs (28 cents) and a free box on the ear. His shop was destroyed in WW II. Since then, he has been cutting hair in a small arbor in the back of his garden in Lübeck. As there is no water, he cuts dry. His granddaughter prefers going to the competition.

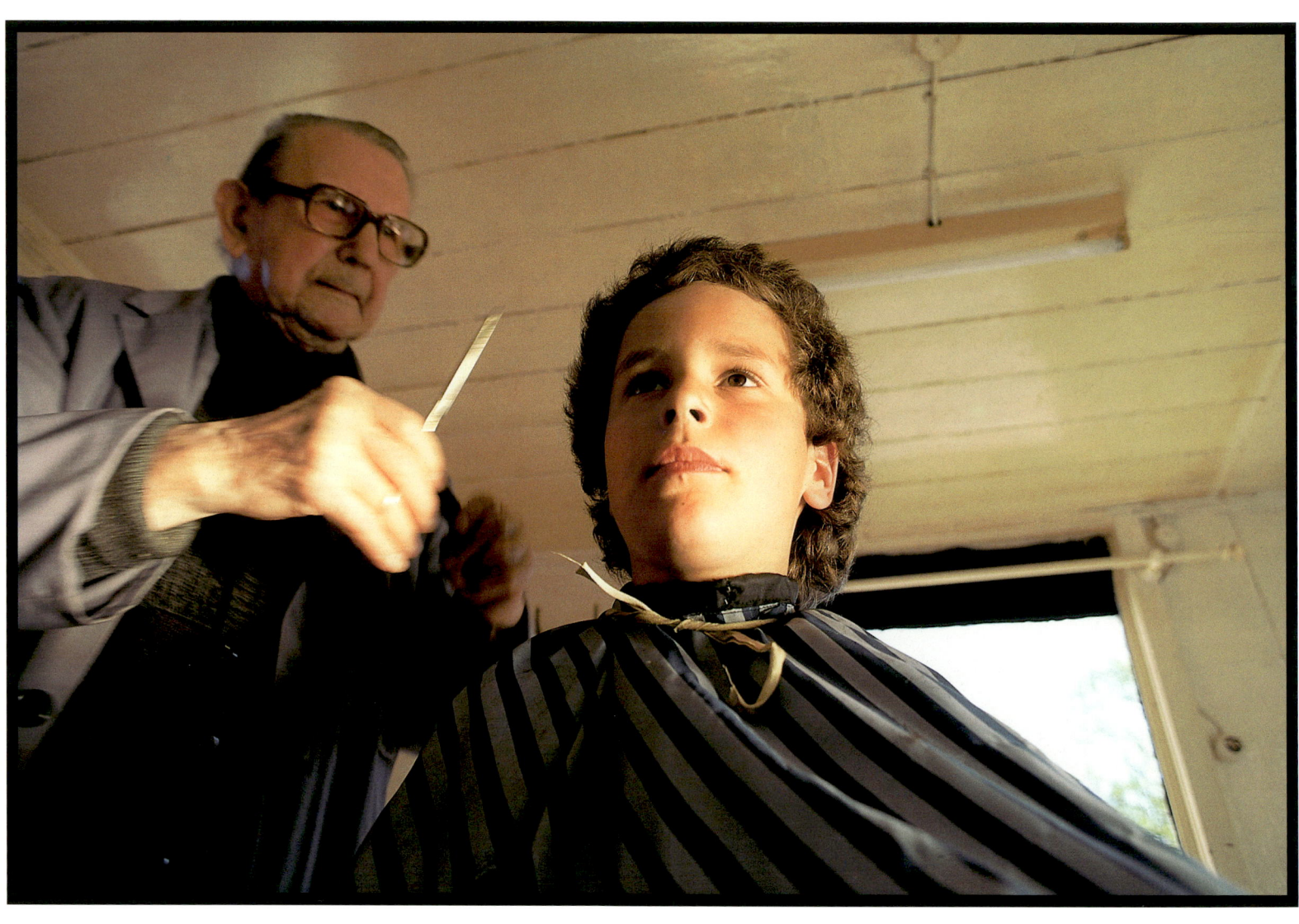

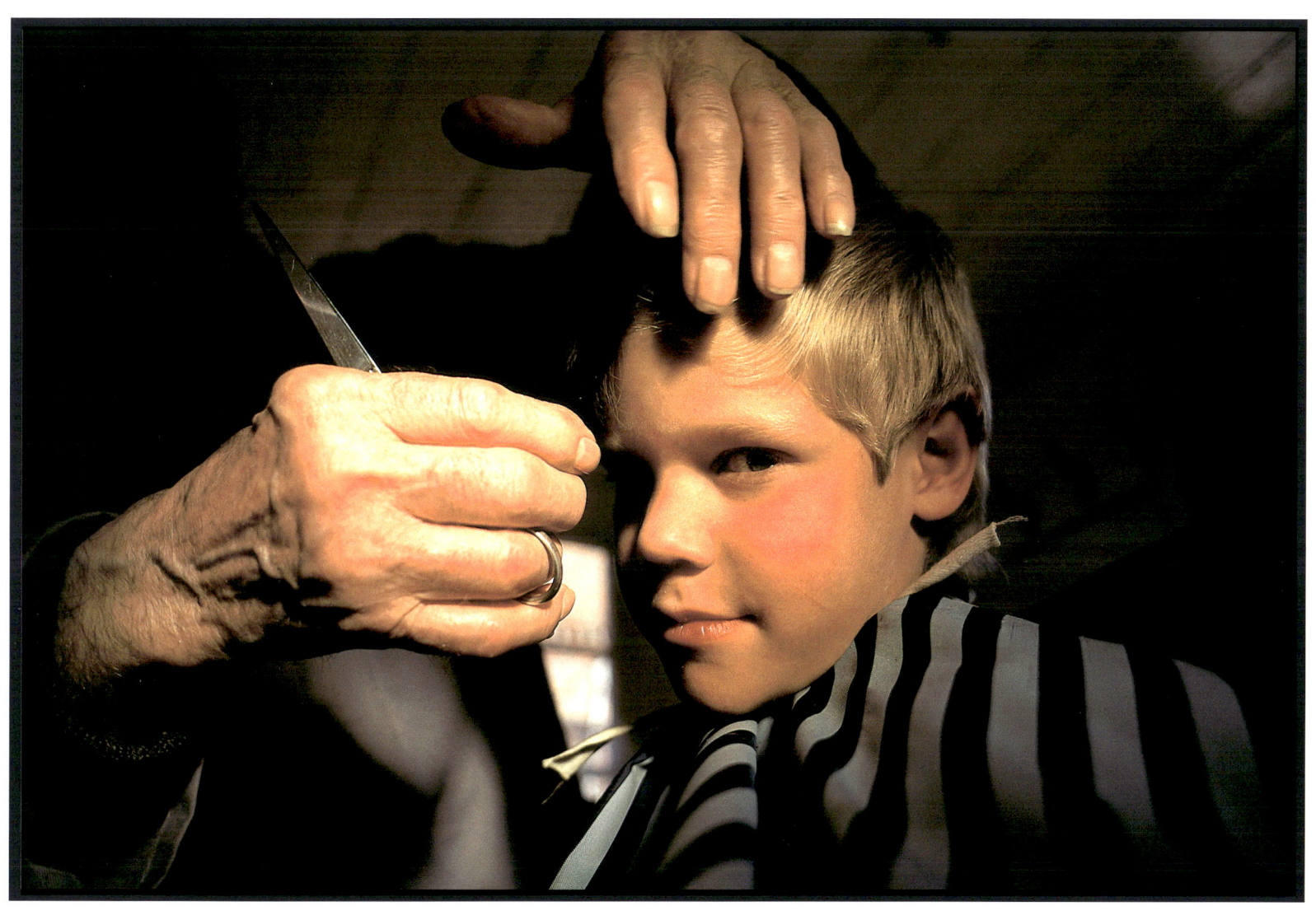

IN BERLIN, the red-maned Valkyrie, Ute Jacobs, organizes occult haircutting sessions with oracles and love potions. Even during the day, metropolitan witches and tigers of the fashionable world feel at home in the theatrical glory of her interior decoration-mix of boudoir, safari or gloomy tomb. Whoever wishes, may have his hair done in an open casket.

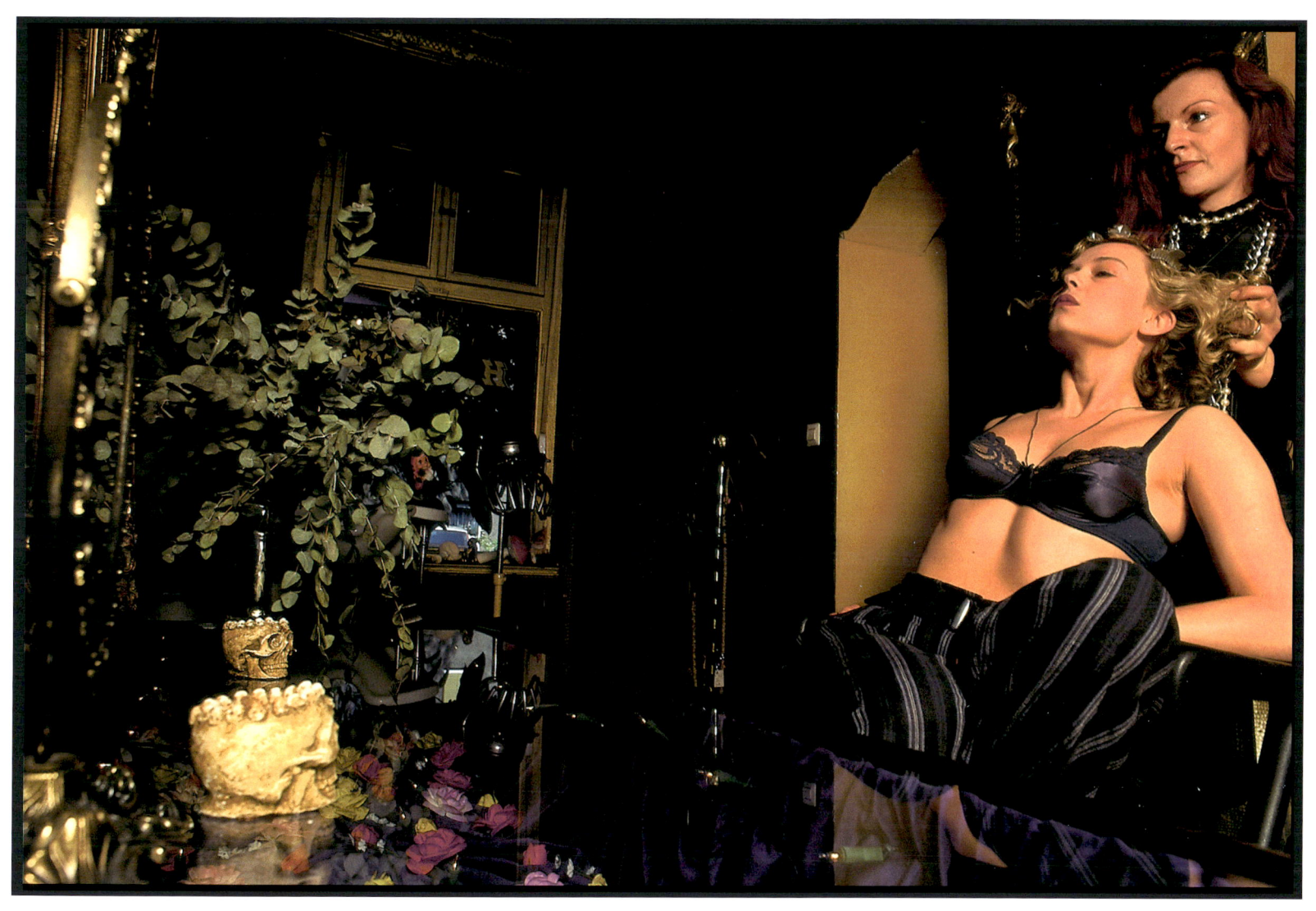

UTE JACOBS/BERLIN

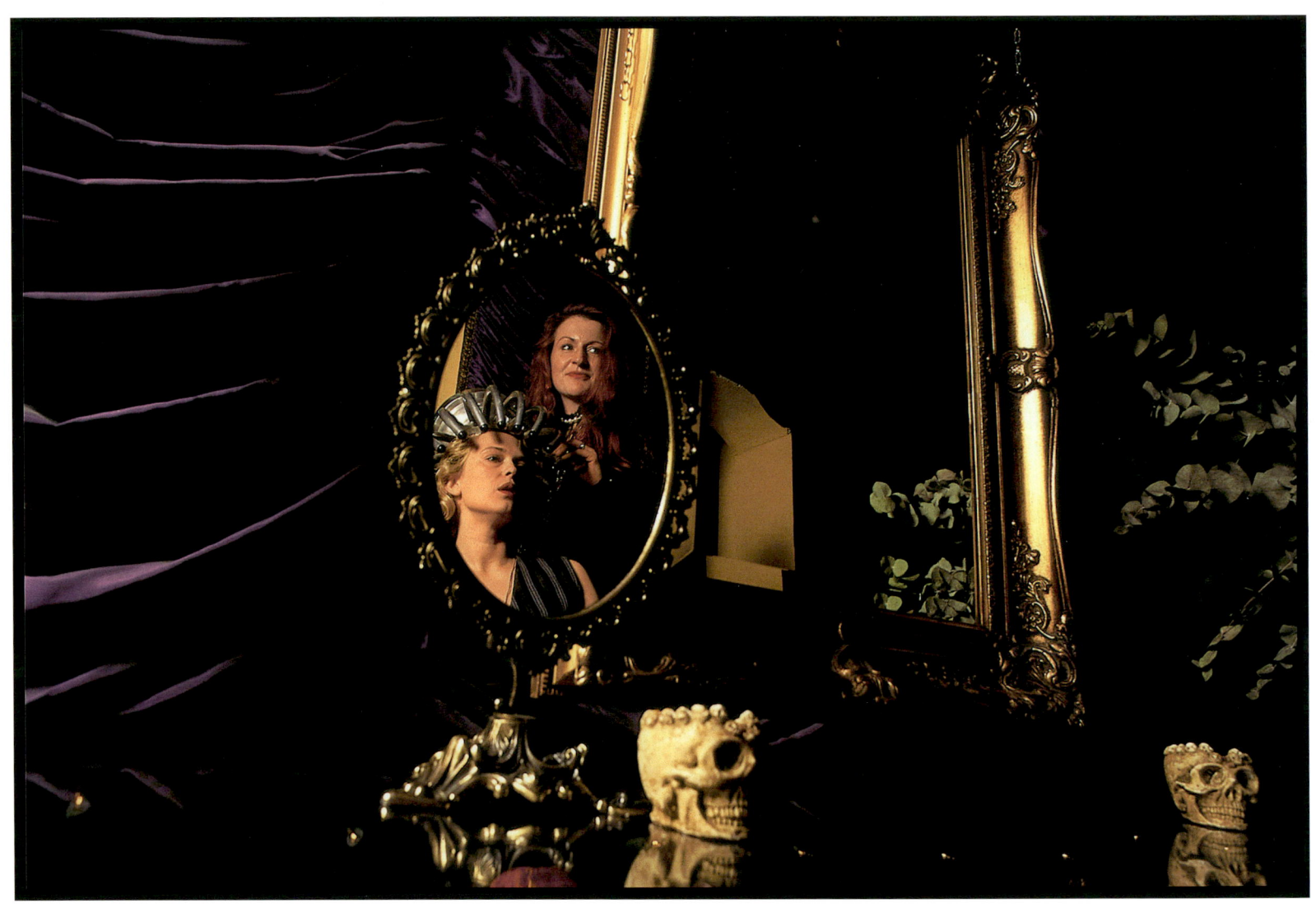

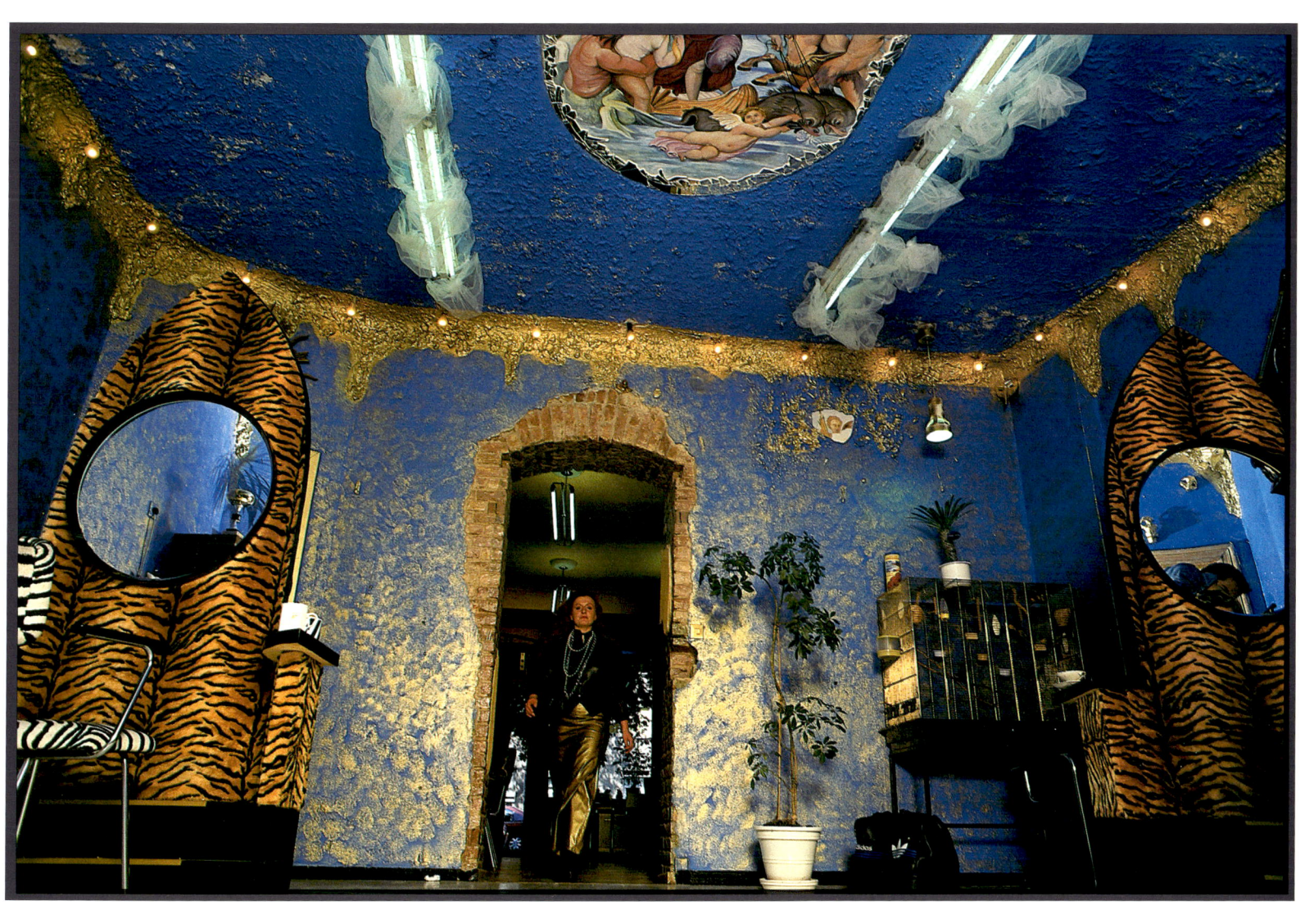

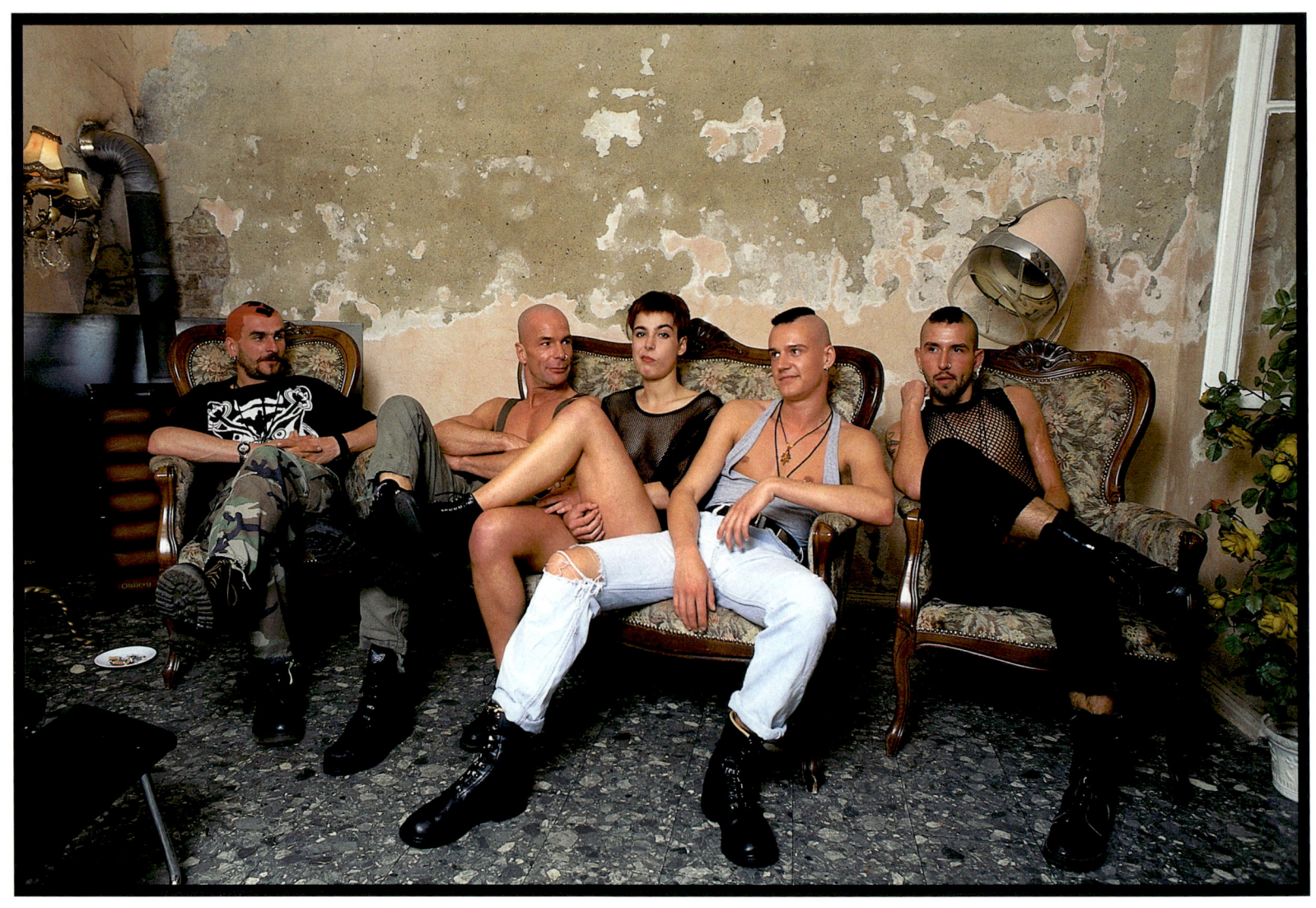

BLOODY CRAFT as in the days of the barber surgeons: nipple-piercing as a special service at a hairdresser's in Berlin-Kreuzberg. Elmar gives the ex-animal caretaker, Mike, the "ultimate sexual kick" with intimate jewelry. Under local anesthesia, the hairdresser stabs his nipples with a cannula and draws a 3 mm (0.12 in) ring of surgical steel through. This isn't Mike's first time. He really gets off on his pierced penis.

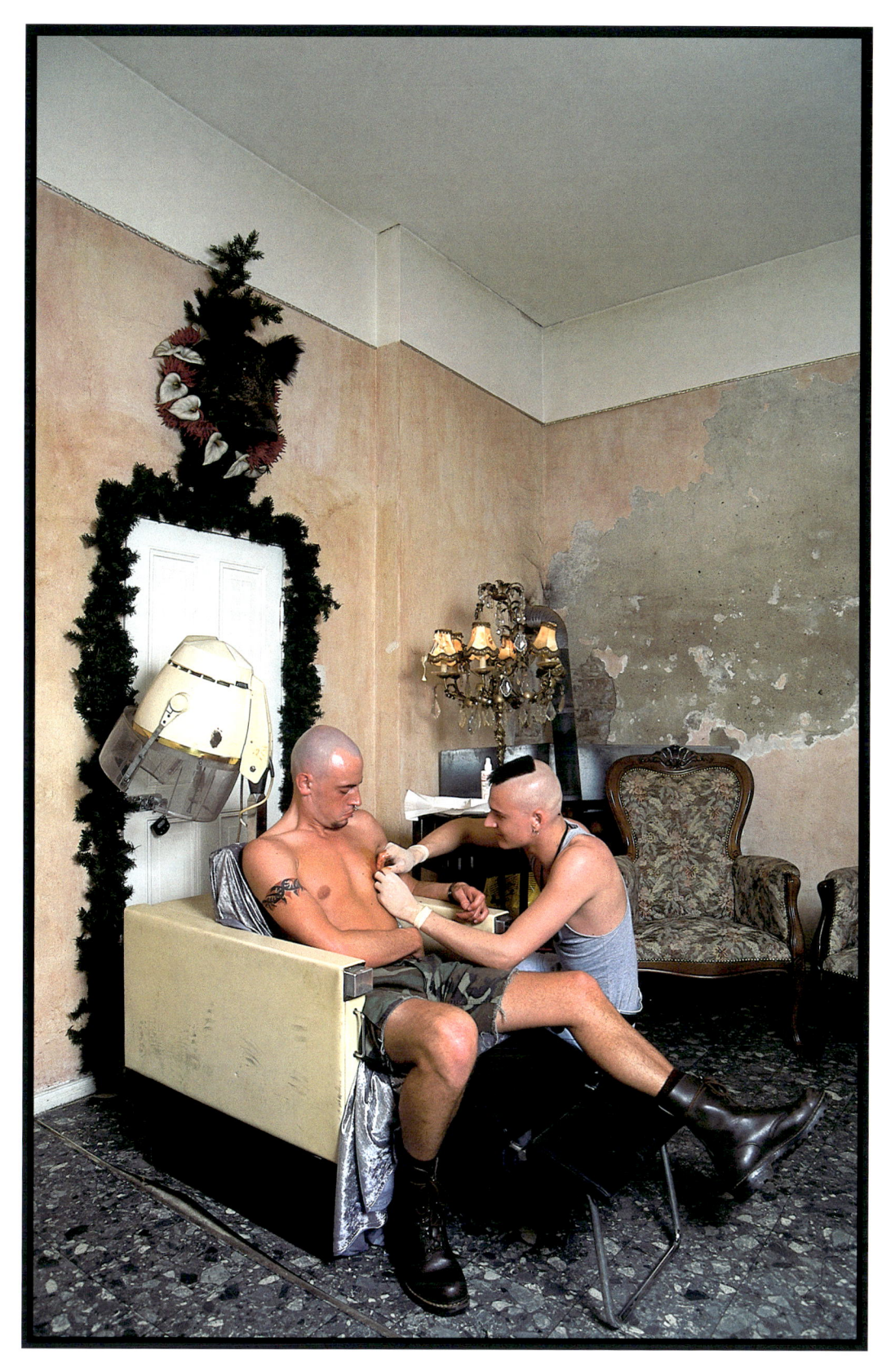

Piercing/Kaiserschnitt, Berlin

HERE YOU CAN BE WHO YOU ARE. In the cozy, home-like environment of her salon in Kassel, Doris Gibonie consoles lonely hearts and serves coffee to accompanying gossip about Europe's royalty, pets, retirement, and grandchildren. An often, a total of 240 years sit in a row, getting perms.

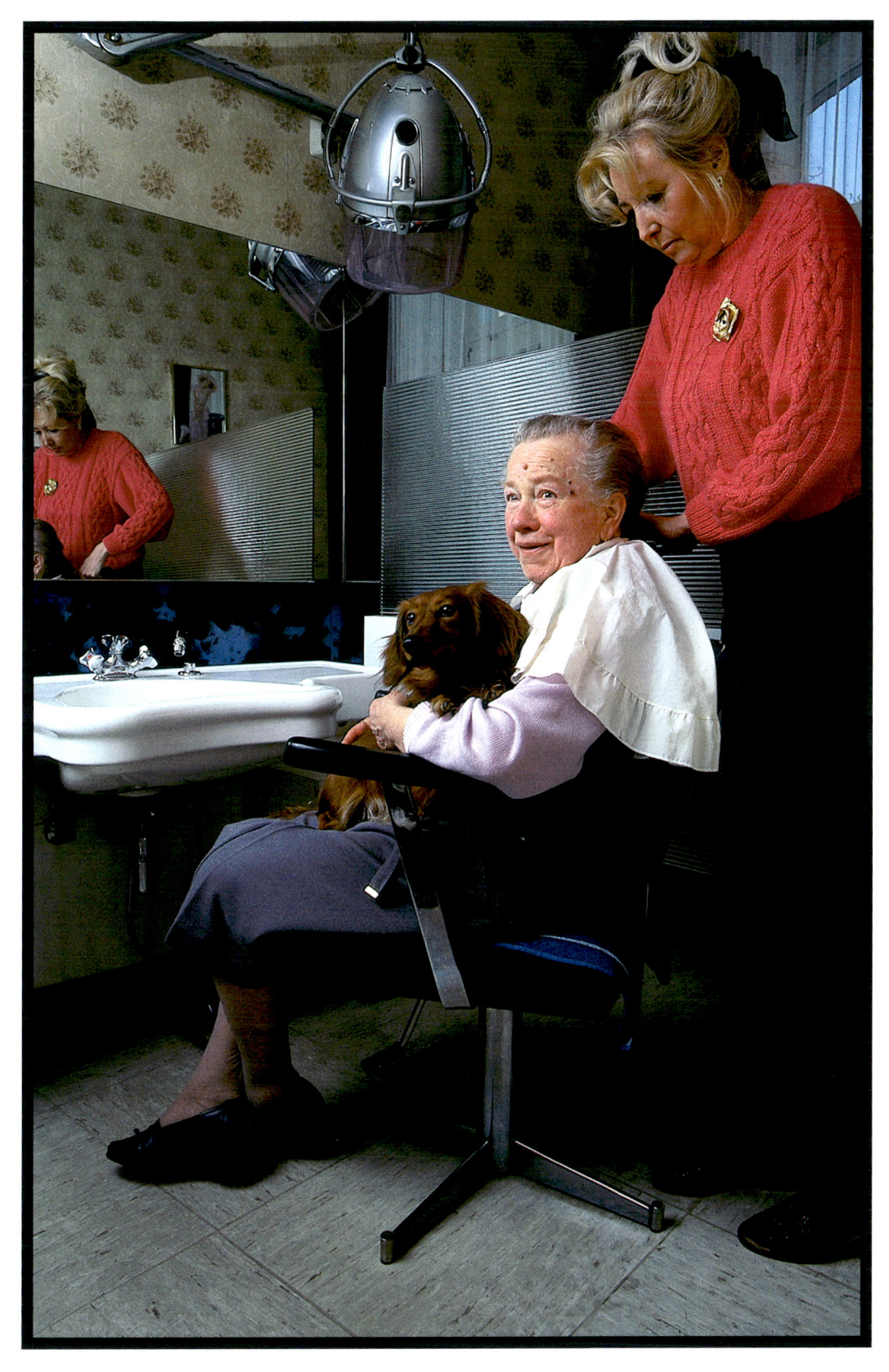

DORIS GIBONIE/KASSEL

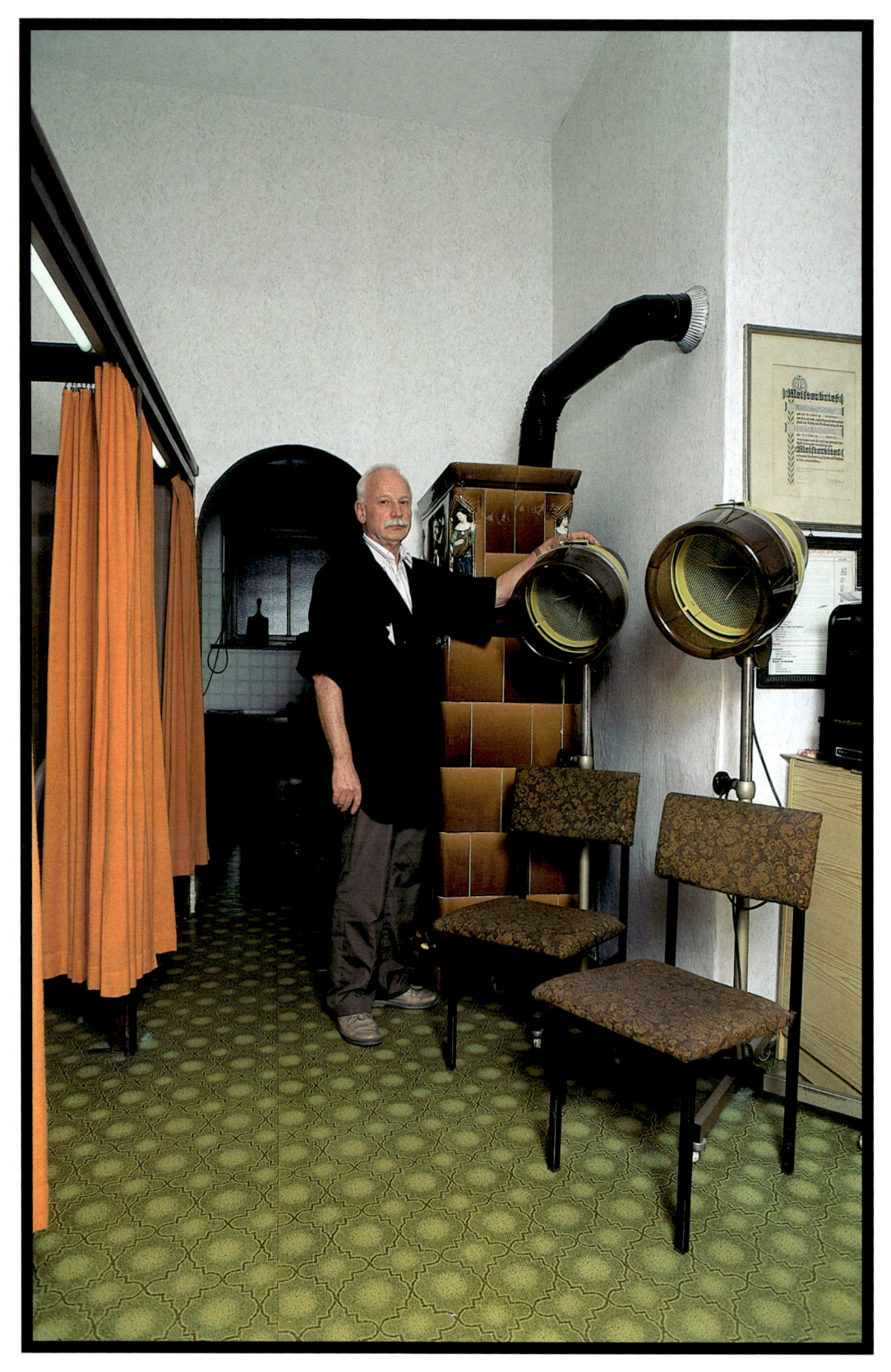

SALON SCHÖNE/MEISSEN

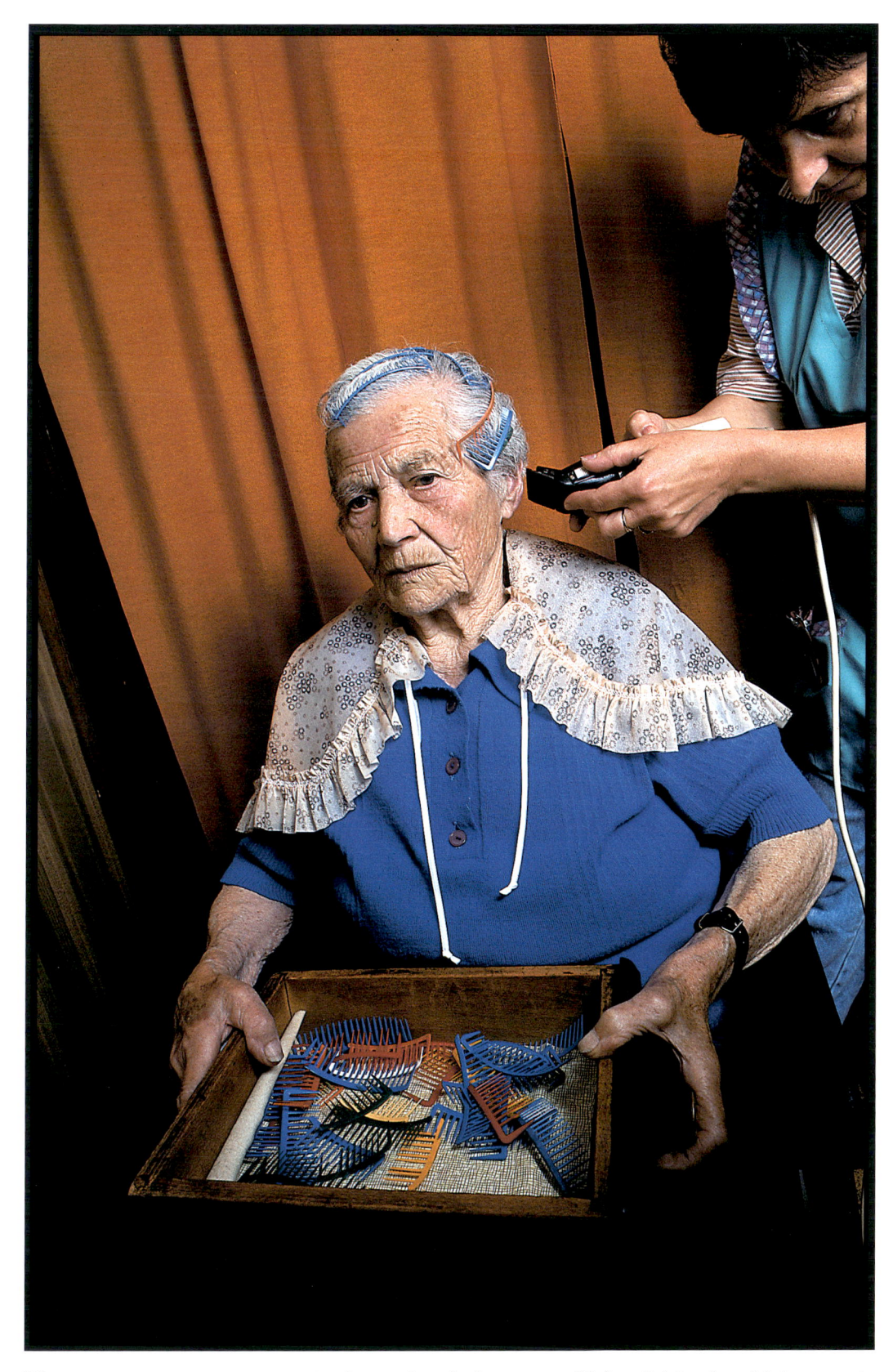

WASHING AND CURLING in front of a tiled stove: at "Salon Schöne" at Meissen train station a loyal customer is being dolled up for the weekend. Blue and red combs bring about the proper pep; the nape is neatly shaven.

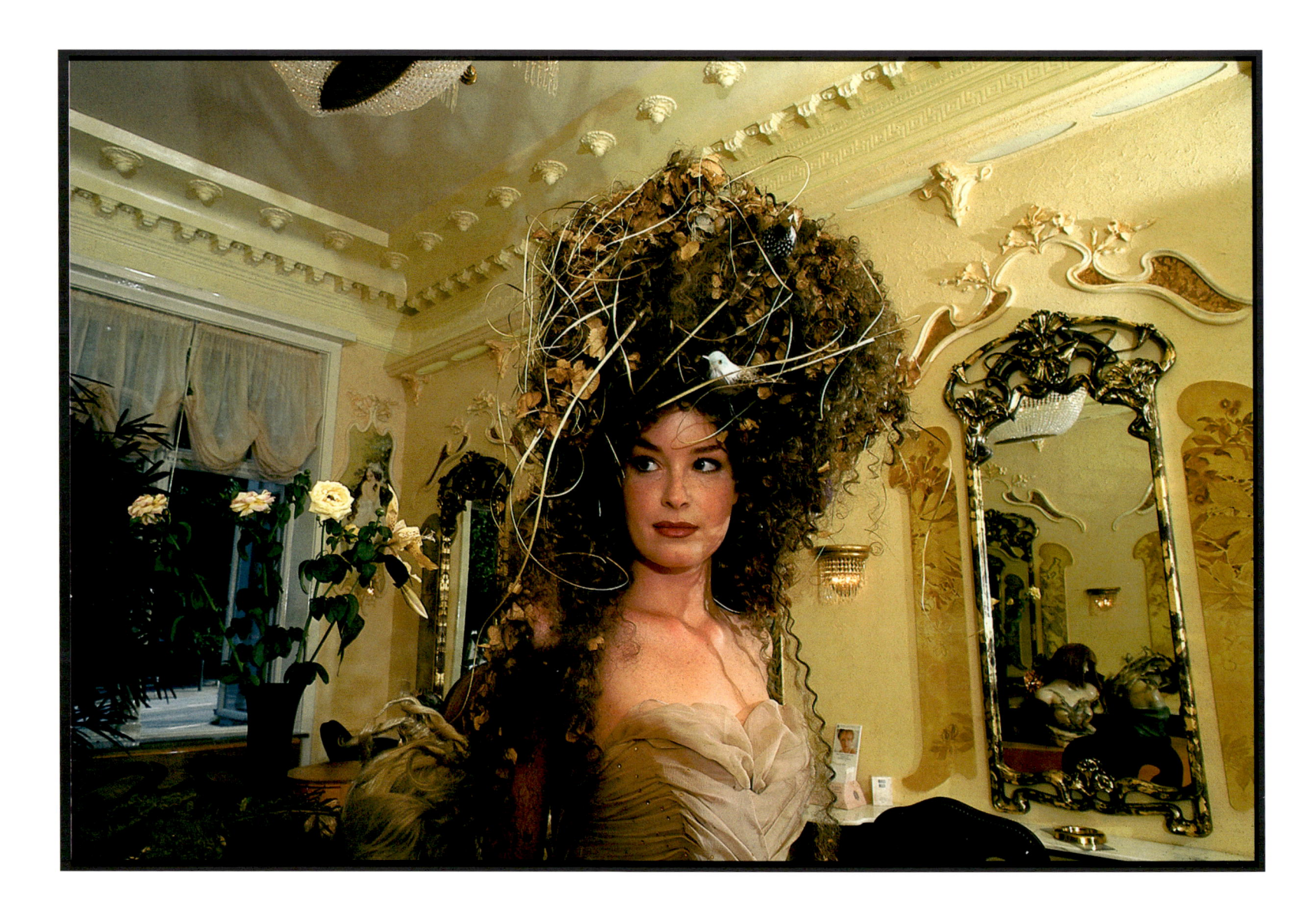

TO HER FANS she is the "Queen Mother of the Branch." Marlies Möller is quite proud to be a trend-setter with international flair. In her beauty-temple, located in an old Hamburg patrician villa, 75 employees wait on some 200 customers daily, many of them celebrities. The busy boss also works as makeup artist and stylist for film and theater, and markets her own line of exclusive haircare products and accessories.

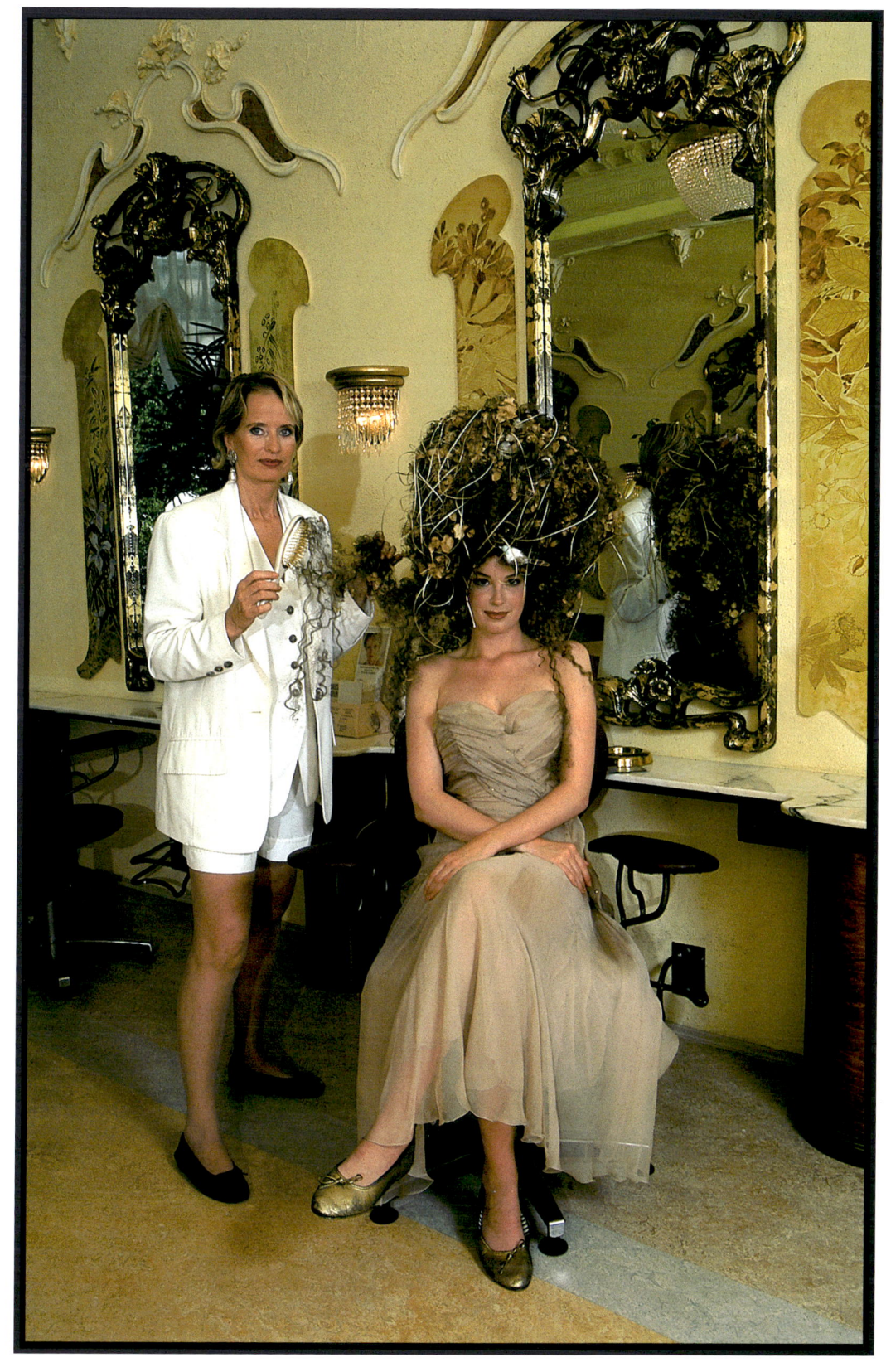

MARLIES MÖLLER/HAMBURG

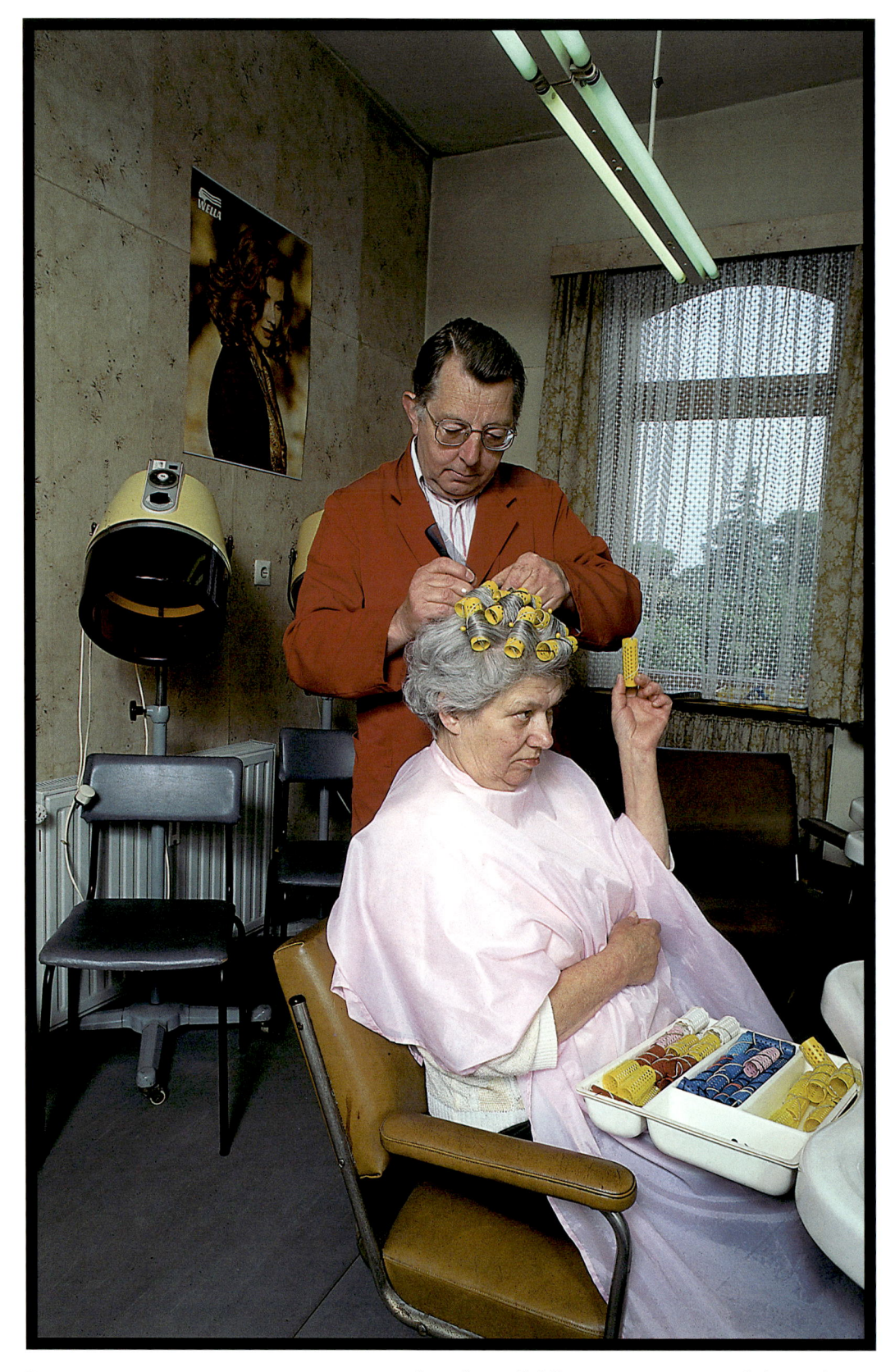

JUST LIKE THE GOOD OLD DAYS: when the wall fell, Henning Kassner did not change a thing in his Meissener shop. He kept his GDR interior, "Egawell" hair-dryers and, of course, his trophy from the GDR Hairdresser's Championship. 1992, the former Hairdresser's Production Cooperative went into private hands.

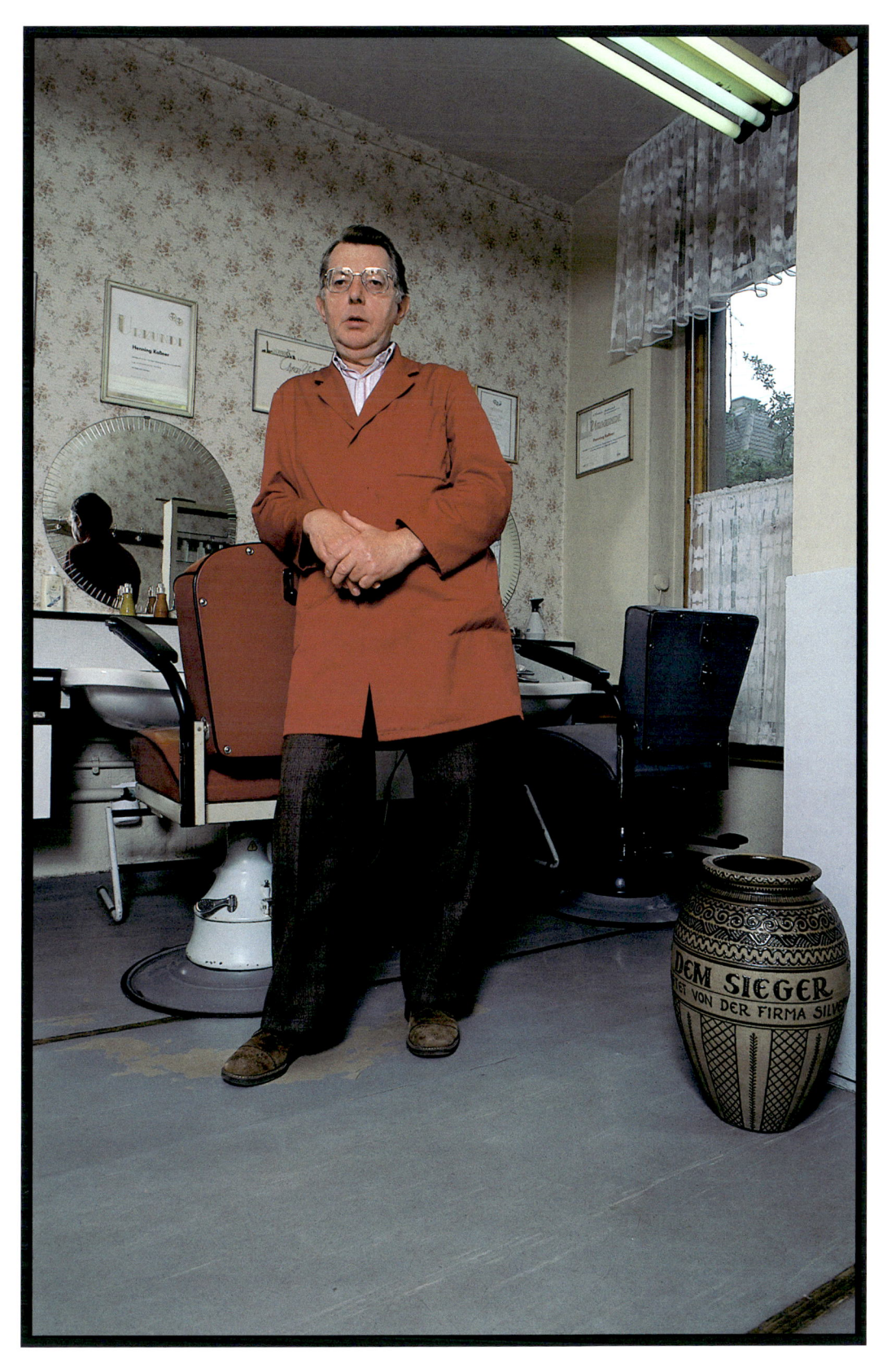

KASSNER/MEISSEN

BARBER, Konrad Babl from Lake Teger near Munich is razor-sharp and definitely no sissy. Martin Schegg has been coming to him for the past 20 years, before he goes to put up the beer tents for the Oktoberfest. In honor of the occasion, Babl gives him a shave and trims his wild mane. Even the local democrats call Babl, who is a fan of Ludwig II, his "Royal Highness." When he gets fed up with the business, this contrary person just closes shop, grabs his gun, and goes hunting chamoix. Babl's master was a licensed barber-surgeon. Fifty years ago, he pulled teeth and did the post-mortem examinations of the deceased in the village.

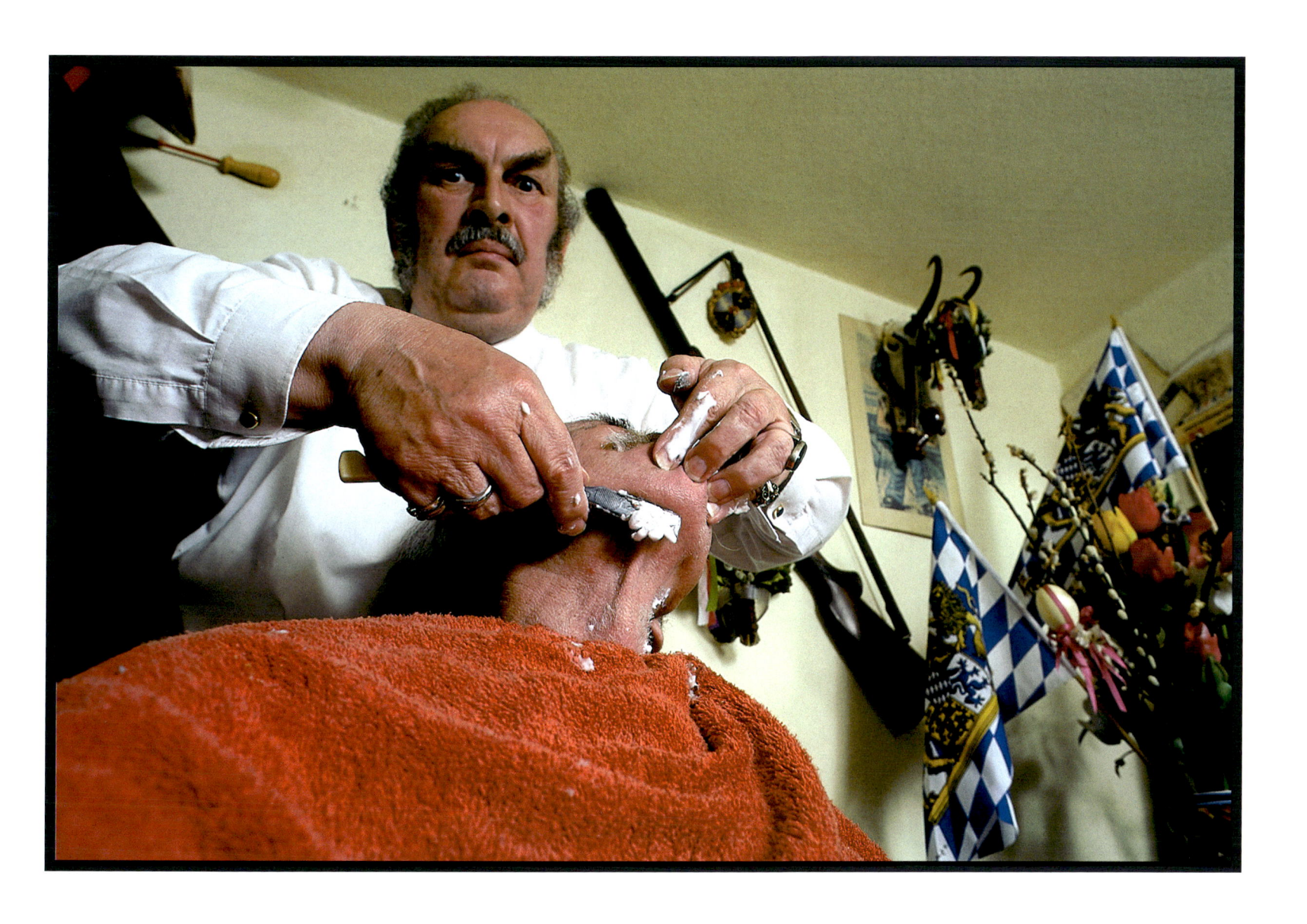

Konrad Babl/Tegernsee

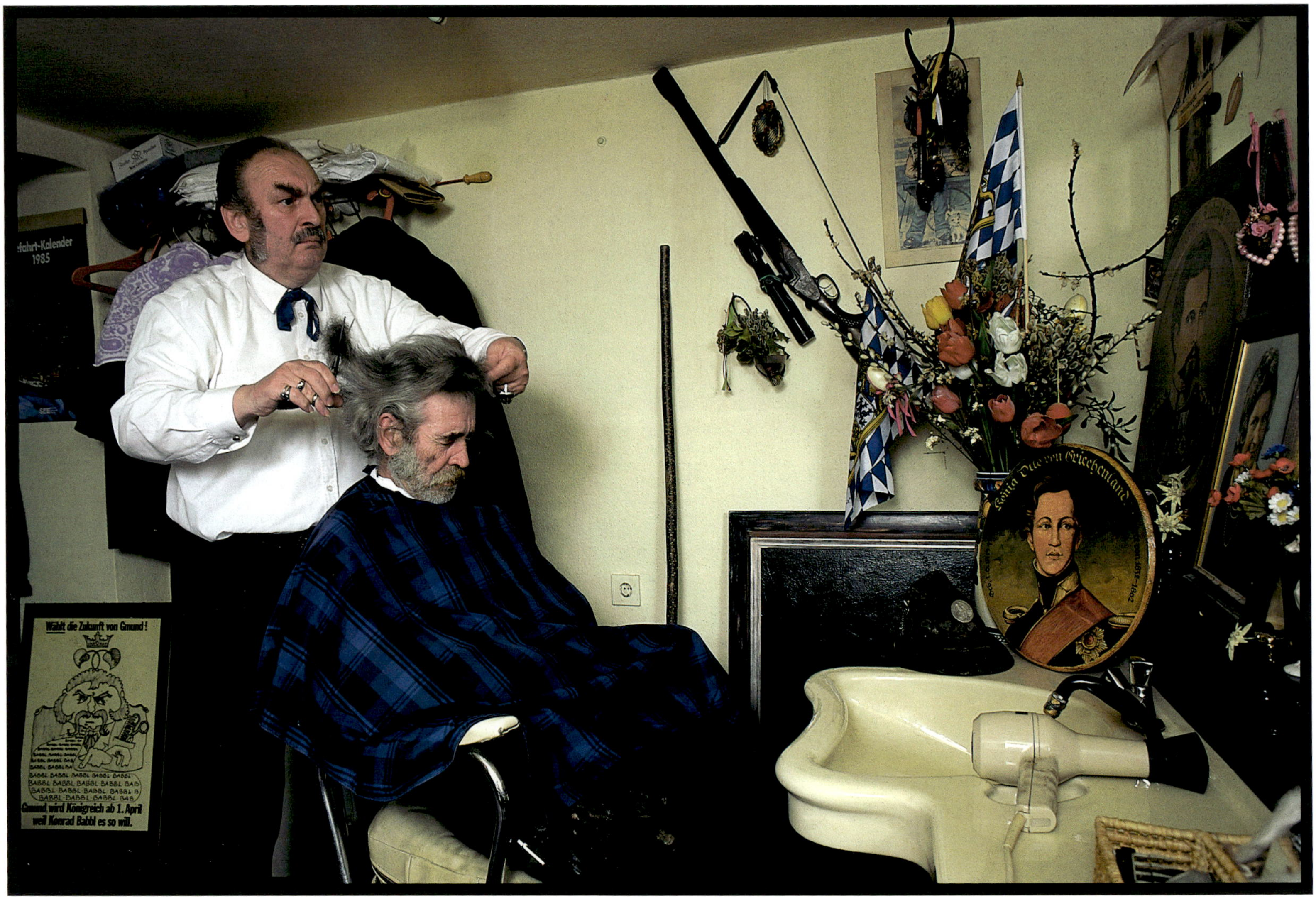
fahrt-Kalender
1985
Wählt die Zukunft von Gmund!
BABBL BABBL BABBL BABBL BABBL
BABBL BABBL BABBL BABBL BAB
BABBL BABBL BABBL BABBL B
BABBL BABBL BABBL BAB
Gmund wird Königreich ab 1. April
weil Konrad Babbl es so will.

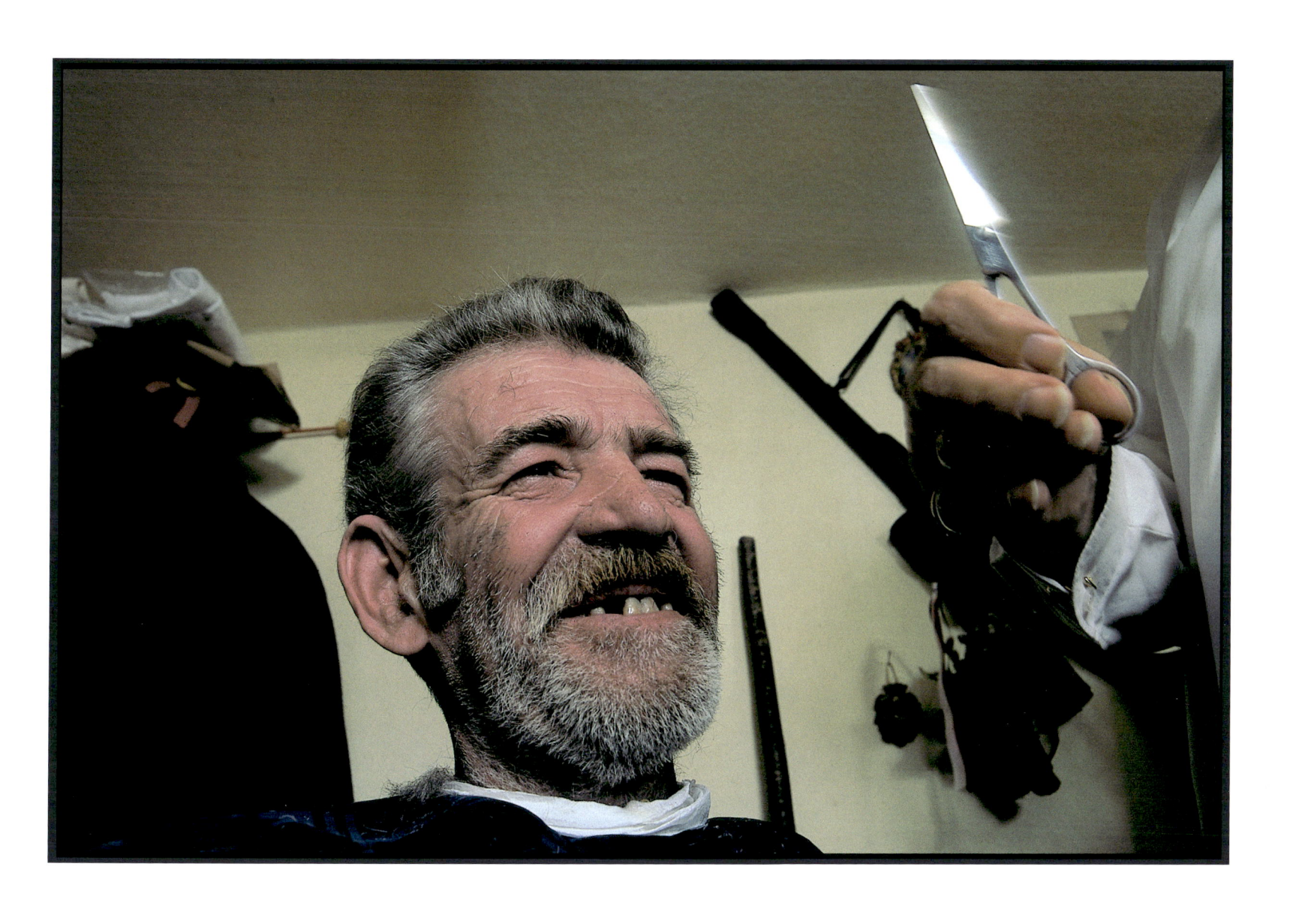

Countess Irina Gräfin Stauffenberg has been a loyal patron of her Figaro Gerhard Meir for ten years. And that despite the fact that the first time she went to his Munich luxury salon "Le Coup" he left her waiting for her perm for a 1920s party for five hours – while half of the party guests sat patiently beside her.

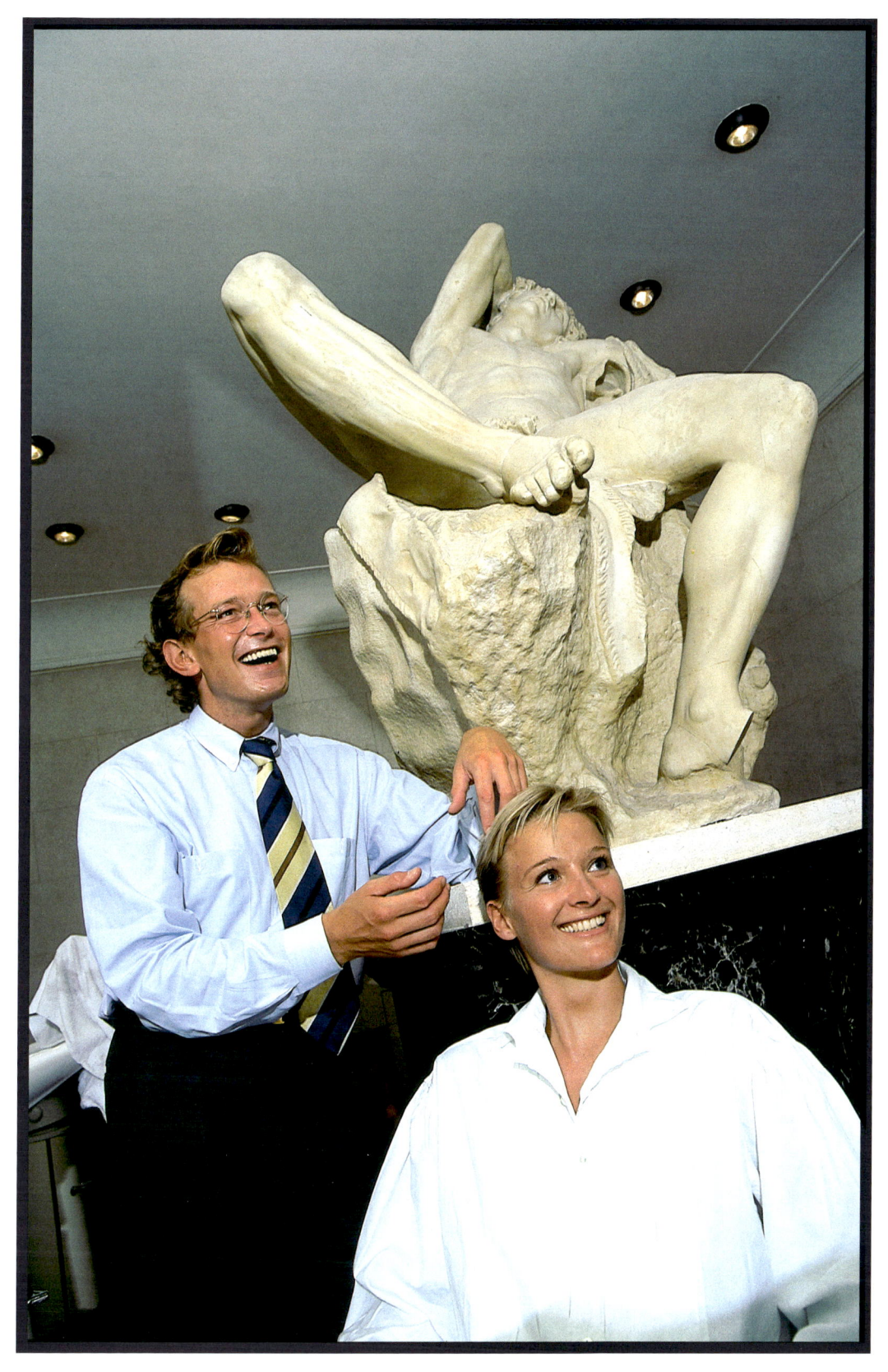

GERHARD MEIR/MUNICH

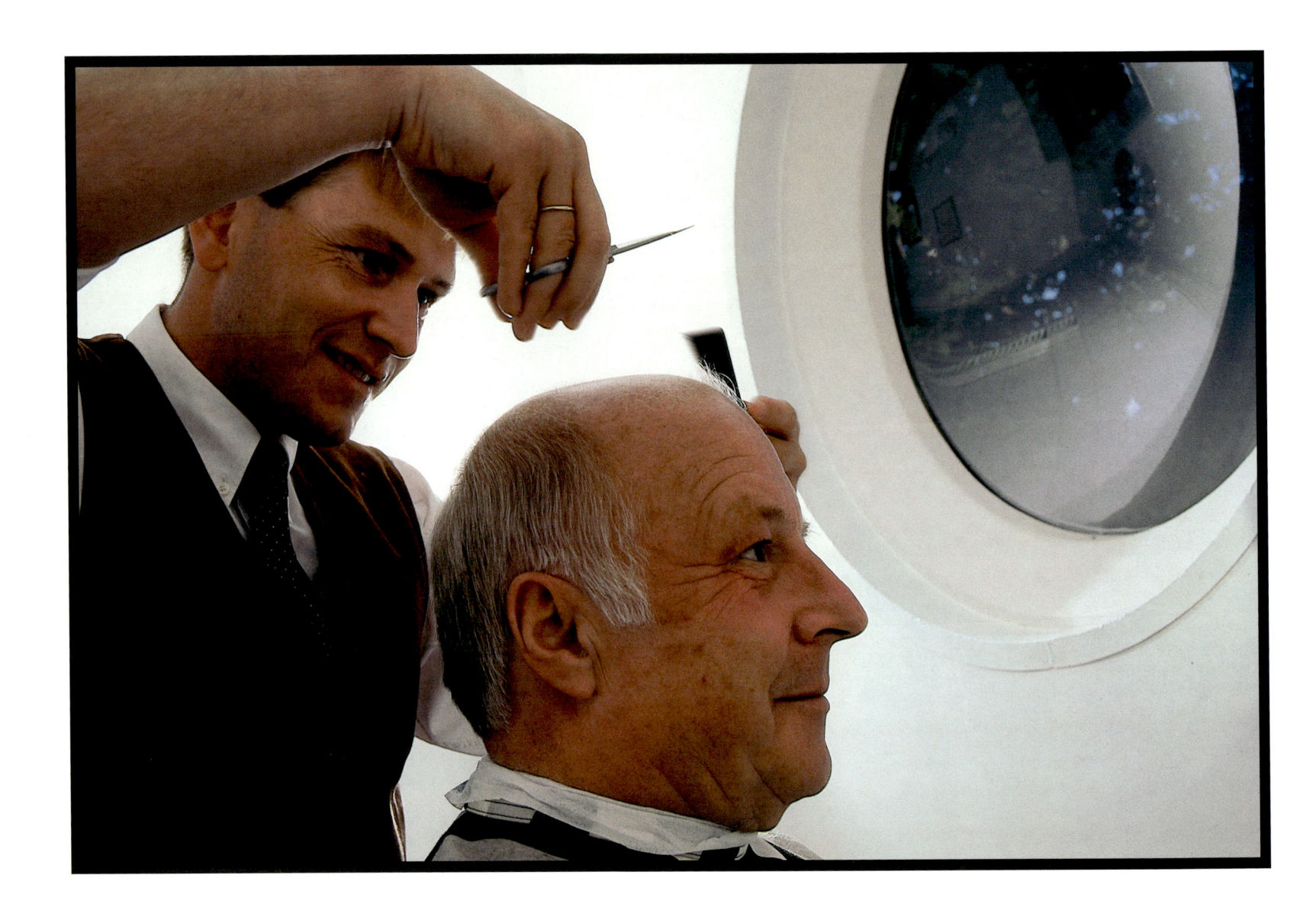

AT PARLIAMENT in Bonn, Norbert Blüm risks his head at the Bundestag hairdresser's. The Federal Minister of Labor pays DM 18 ($ 10) to have his hair cut by Udo Münch. The séparé with its simple interior and port-hole view of the Rhine is also available to Chancellor Kohl.

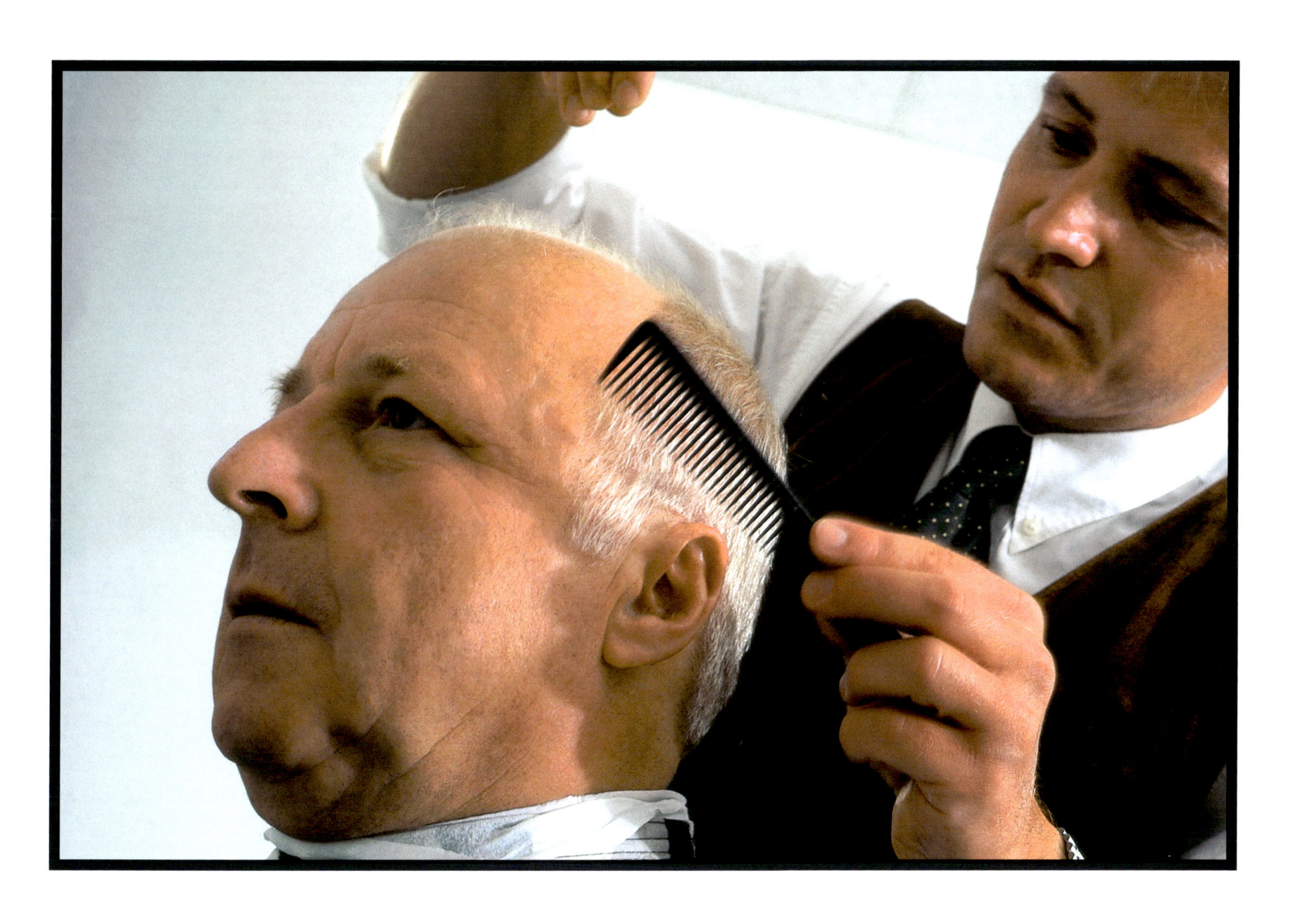

BUNDESTAG HAIRDRESSER MÜNCH/BONN

In "Sikrodil," a red stalactite cave in Munich, owner Siggi Einmeier creates braided hair-dos with 65 cm-long (26 inches) genuine hair strands. The six-hour-procedure seals the false splendor with a special wax for six months. The customer has to dole out a hefty DM 600–800 ($ 333–444). Globe-trotter Siggi named her unusual salon after an adventurous encounter with a bite-happy crocodile.

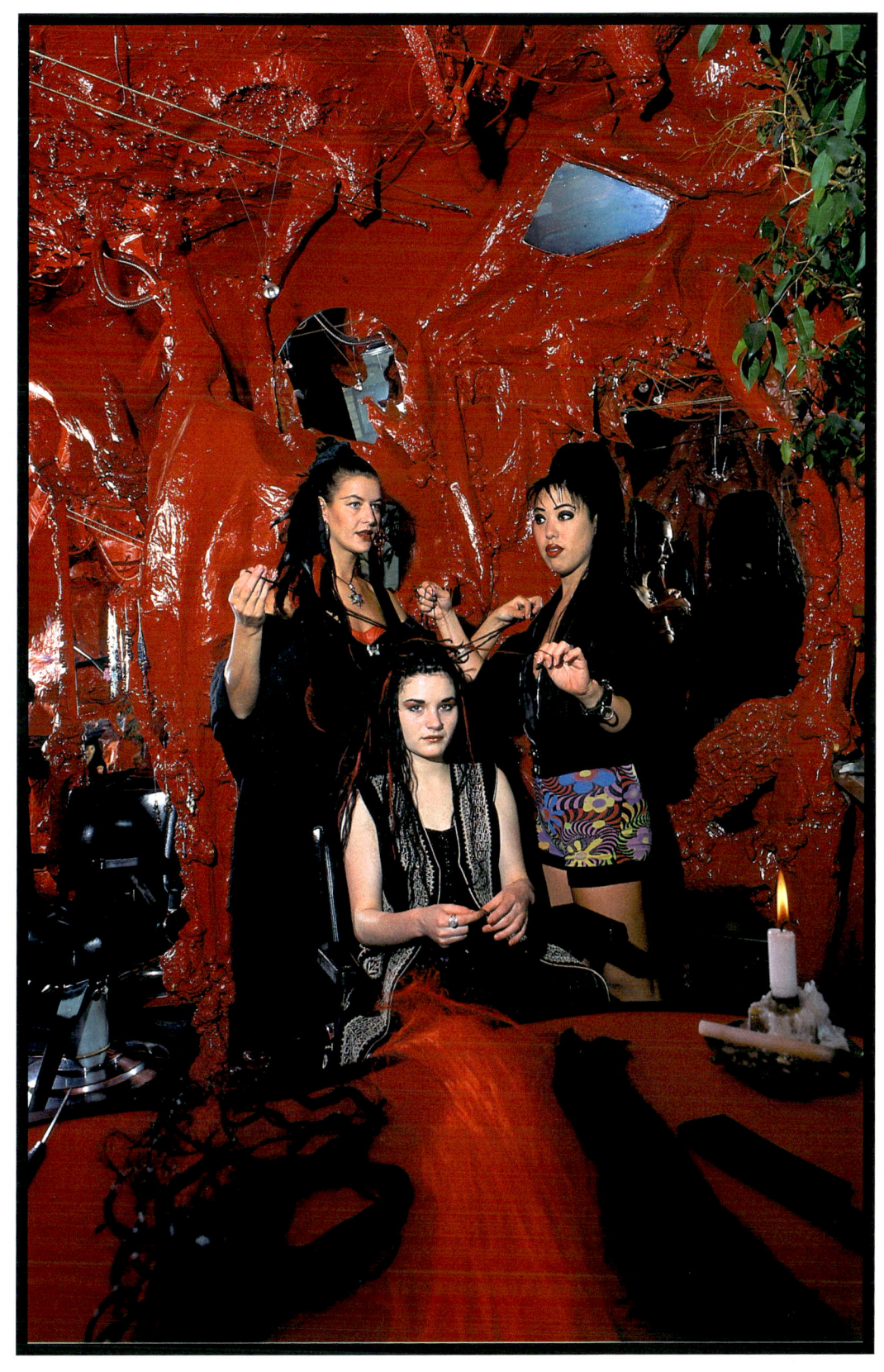

SIKRODIL/MUNICH

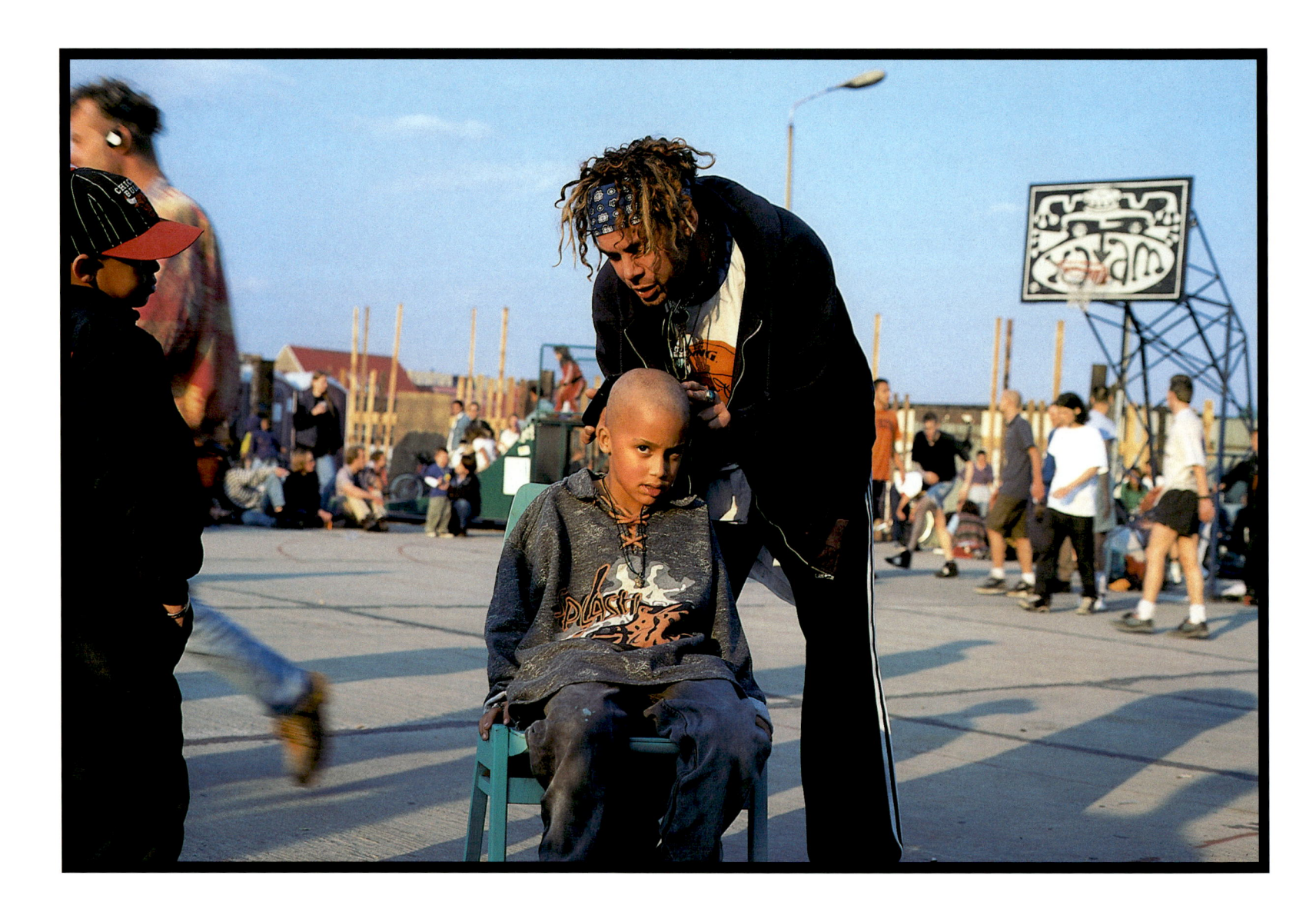

NOT ONLY does Jonny Pazzo from Berlin let his hair down in his salon "Venus": during a streetball tournament, at the edge of the players' field, he shaves Magae's head bald. The Figaro has redone heads of various celebrities. When necessary, he also calls upon the power of crystals: an amethyst on the forehead is supposed to ward off evil seducers and purify the soul.

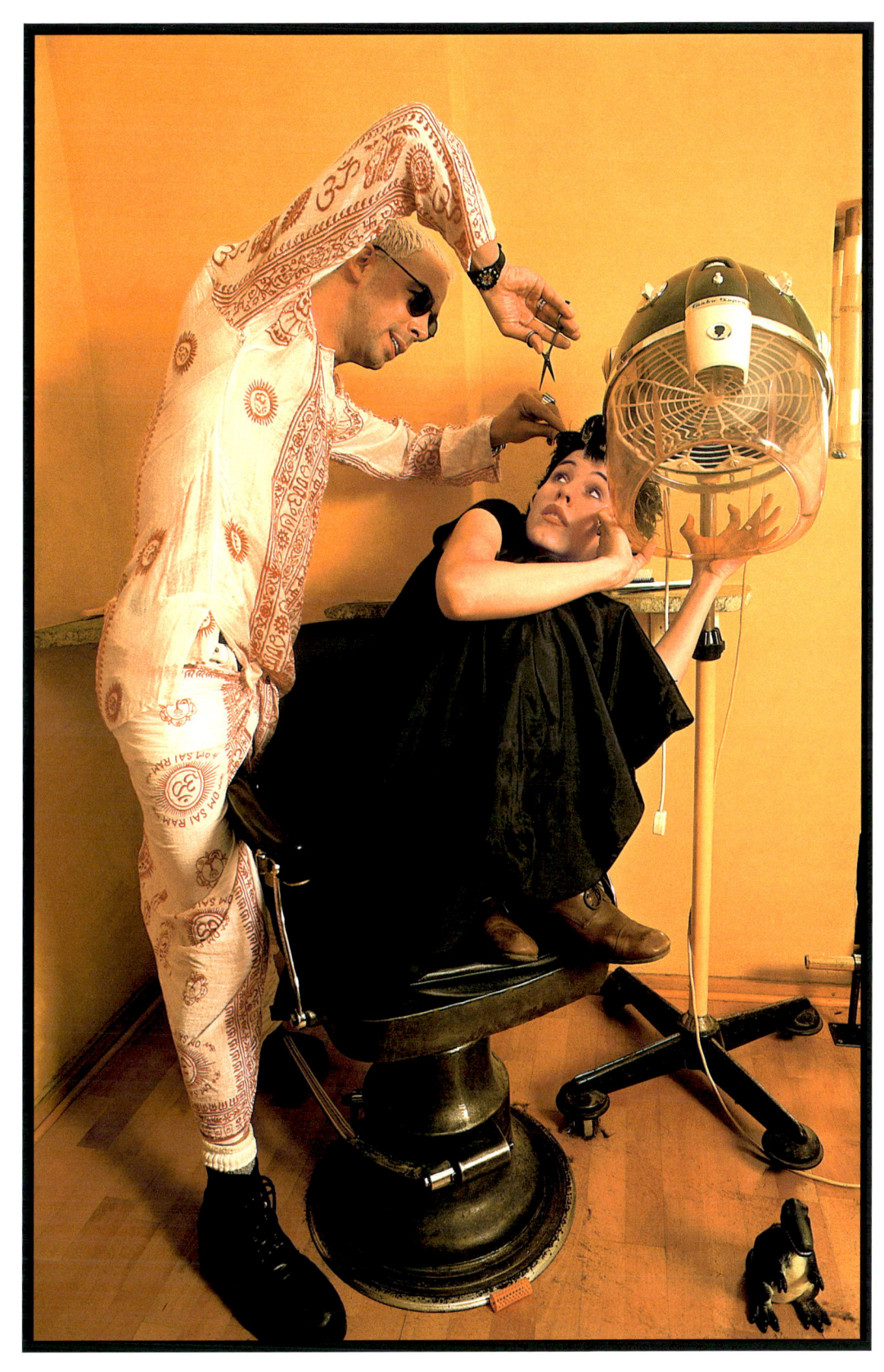

JONNY PAZZO/BERLIN

THE FASHIONABLE salon "Klier" in the stylish Kö-Gallery offers its customers a special service. The stress-plagued may tank up under an oxygen-oasis and bed their weary bodies on a massage armchair, where they relax to celestial tunes and are massaged electrically.

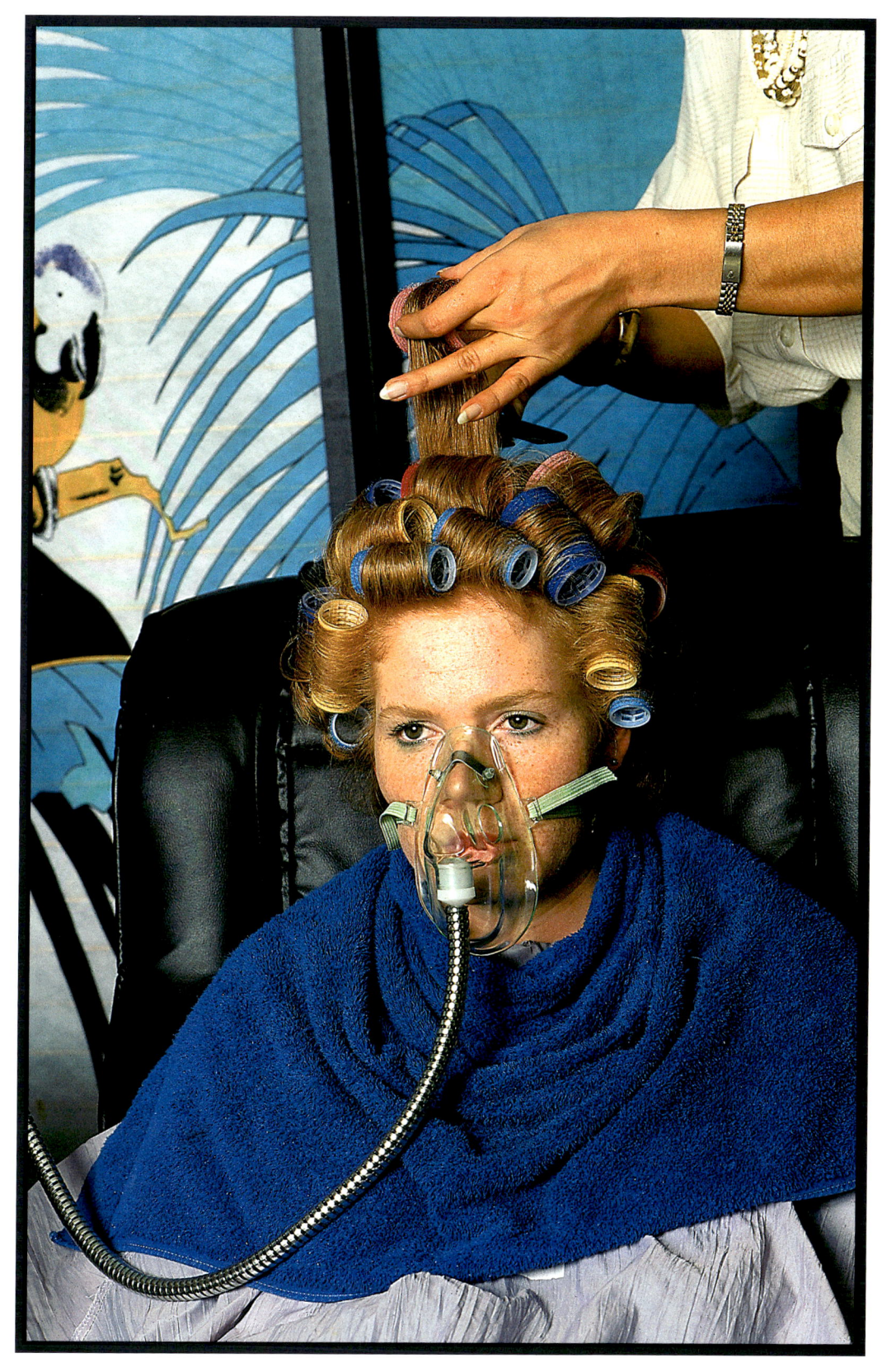

KLIER/DÜSSELDORF

REPORT for hair roll-call at the German Army's barracks in Arolsen. The days of the hair net are over; recruits are having their hair cut short again. On weekends, there is quite a rush for the barber's. Then, the master does assembly-line cutting.

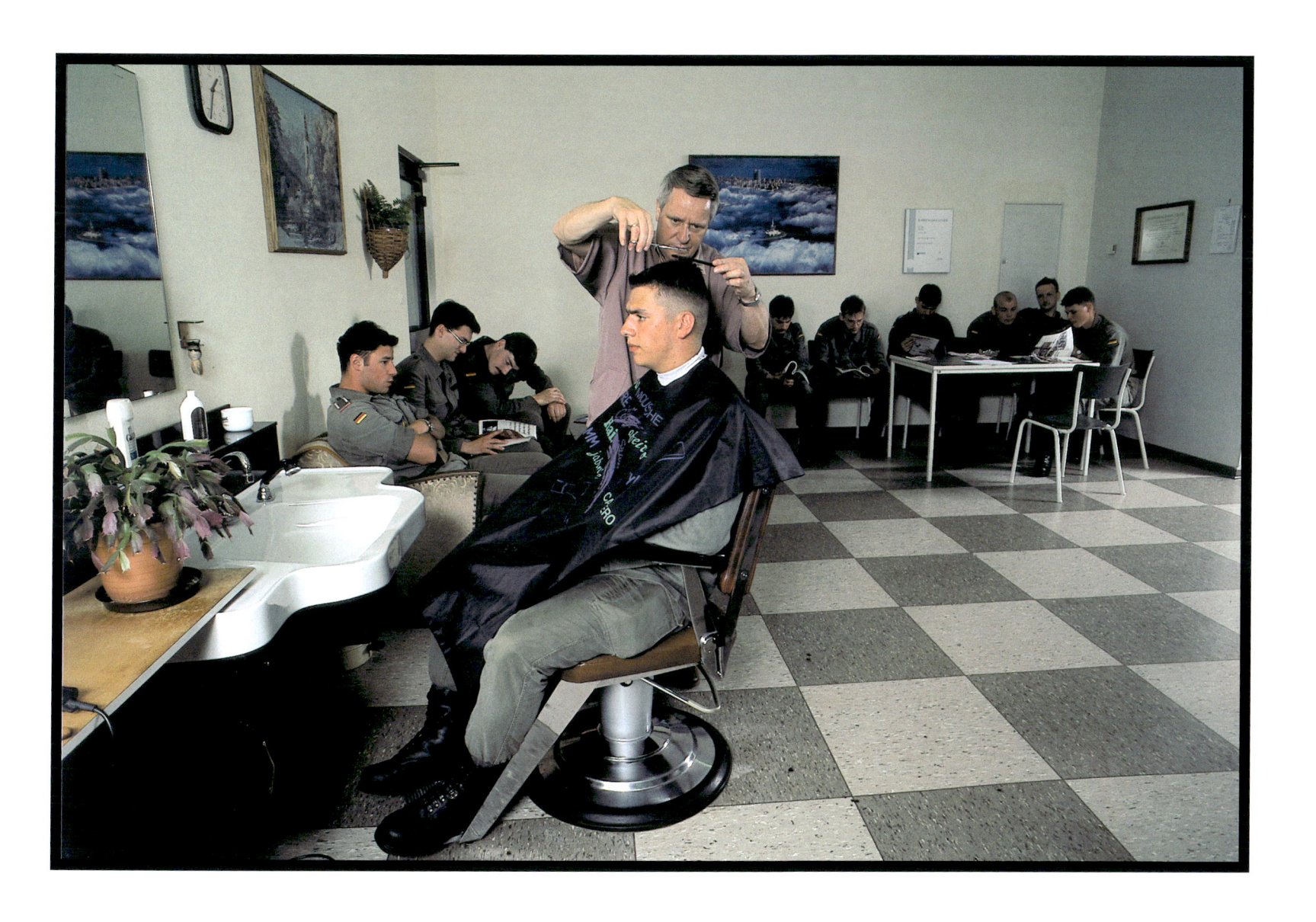

GERMAN ARMY HAIRDRESSER/AROLSEN

AT SCHLOSSHOTEL Bühlerhöhe in the Black Forest, beauty farm and hairdresser's salon are combined. Apart from the exclusive atmosphere, guests enjoy a dream-view of the Black Forest. When the weather is nice, they are styled out on the terrace.

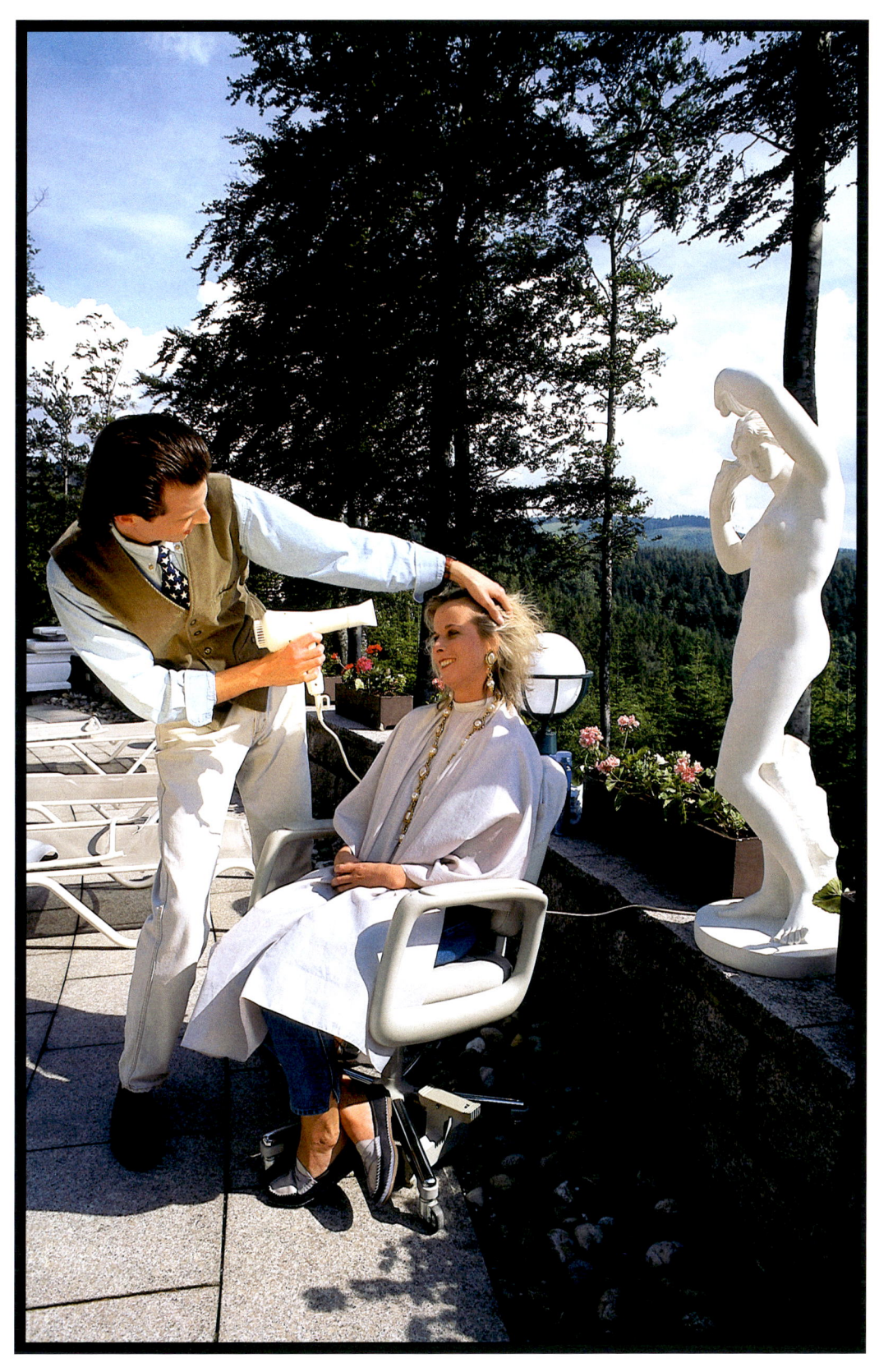

Bühlerhöhe/Black Forest

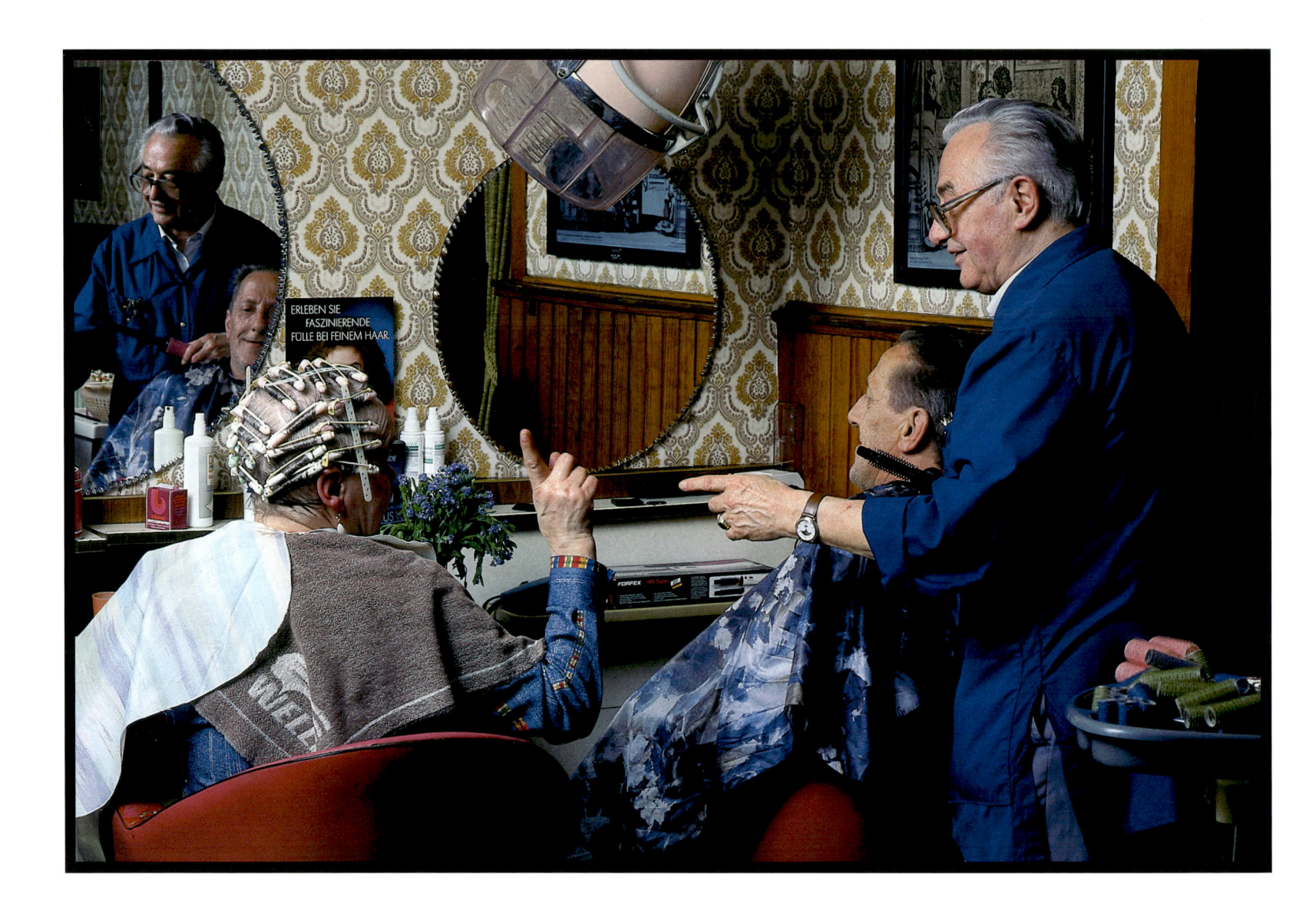

USCHI, who runs "Eulenklause," and her friend "Nose"-Paul meet for a little chat, while hairdresser Thiemann from Hamburg-Ottensen gives her a permanent and him a traditional cut.

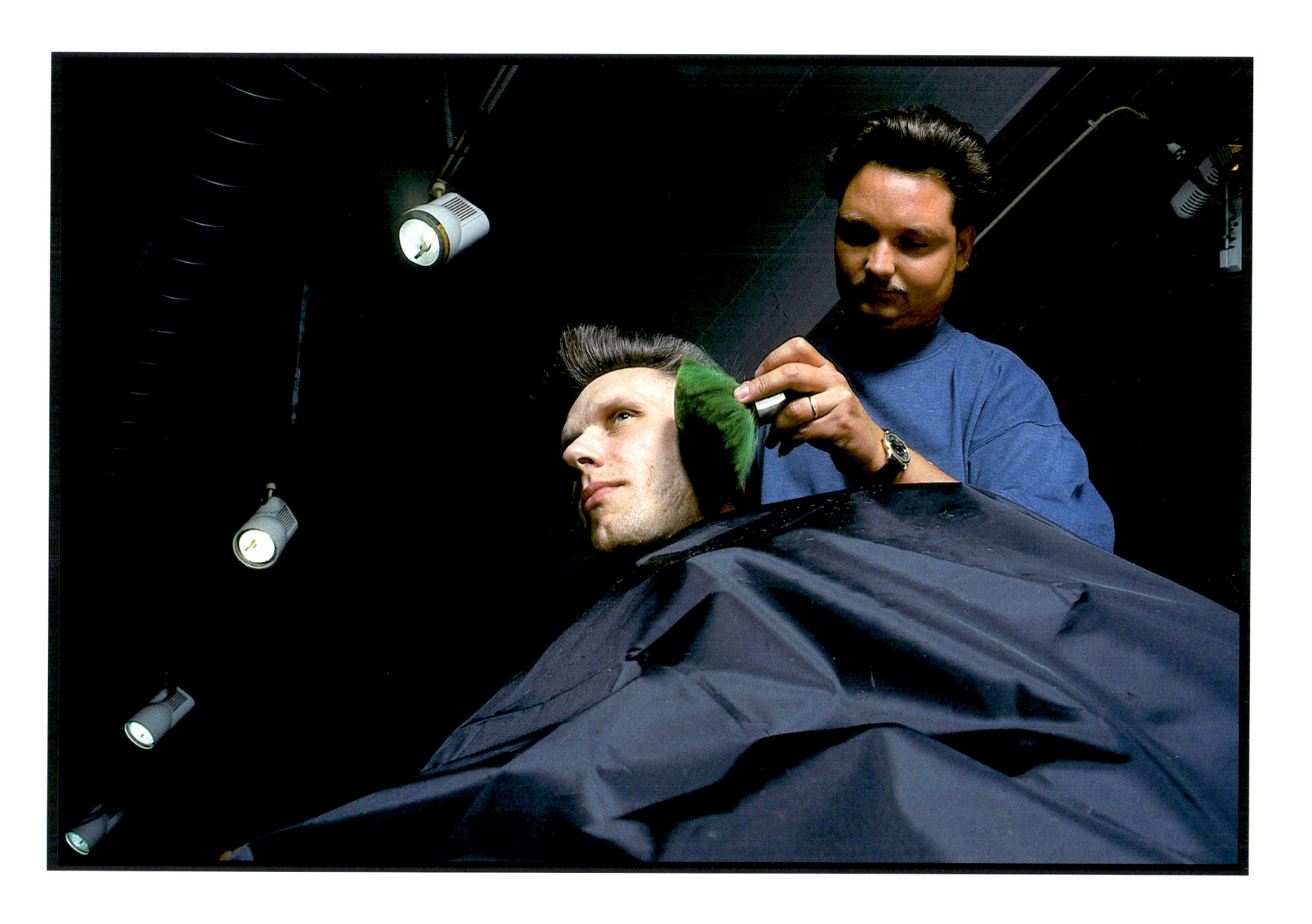

HANS KIPPEL from Bochum panelled his salon "Lettuce" all on his own, using corrugated iron from Brazil. His clientele loves his technical touch: mirrors hang from construction-scaffolding and his speakers boom to a deafening techno-beat.

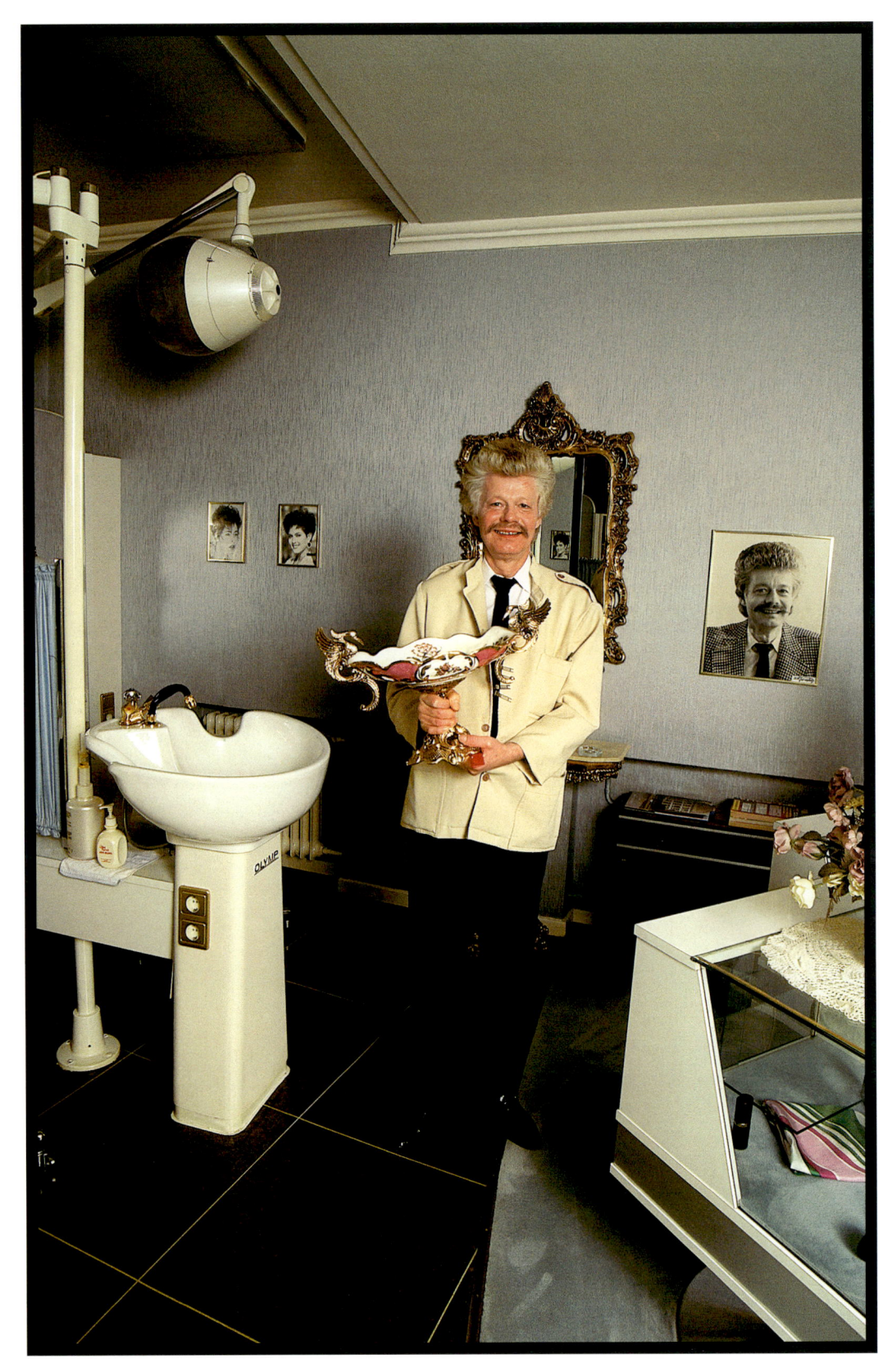

FAHRENHOLZ/BREMEN

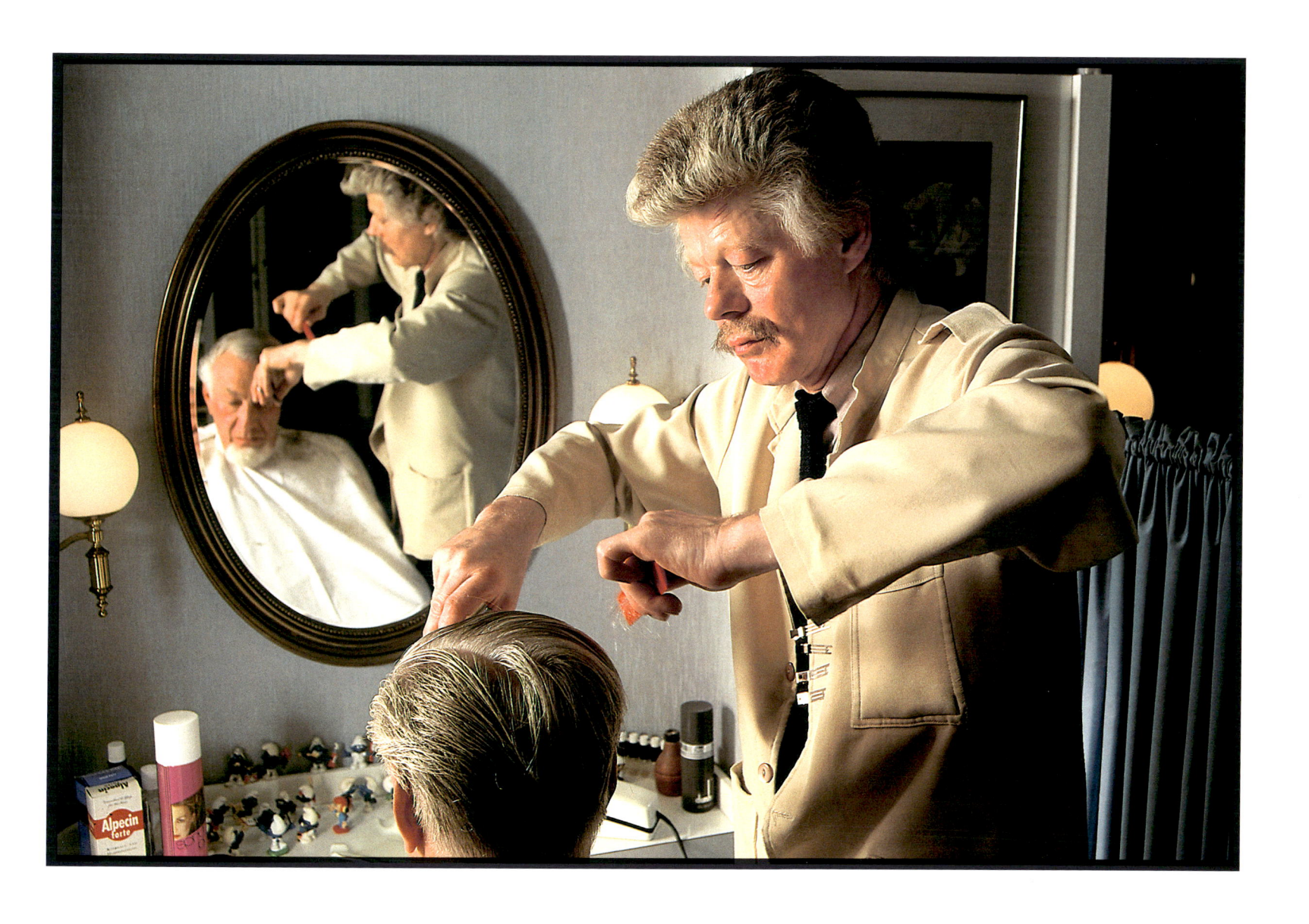

FIGARO Fahrenholz from the "Bremer Parkhotel" dries and sprays until every stubborn hair surrenders to the maestro's sense of order. The boss even combs the fringe of the rugs and brushes the carpets neatly. The porcelain-trophy is his great pride.

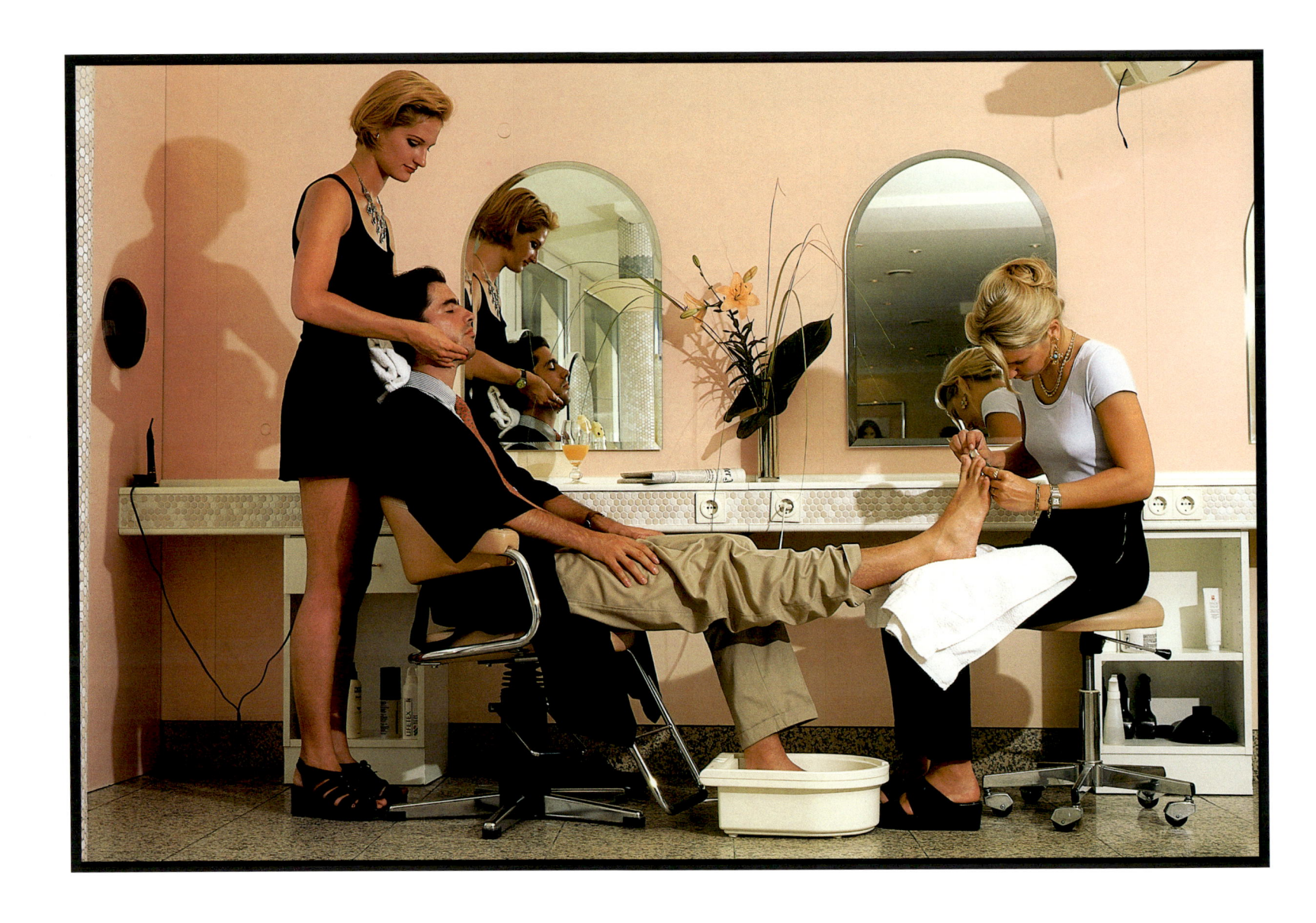

YOUNG stress-plagued managers and bankers love to relax at Ingrid Klee's Frankfurt Salon from marathon meetings and stock-market depression with a pedicure or facial massage.

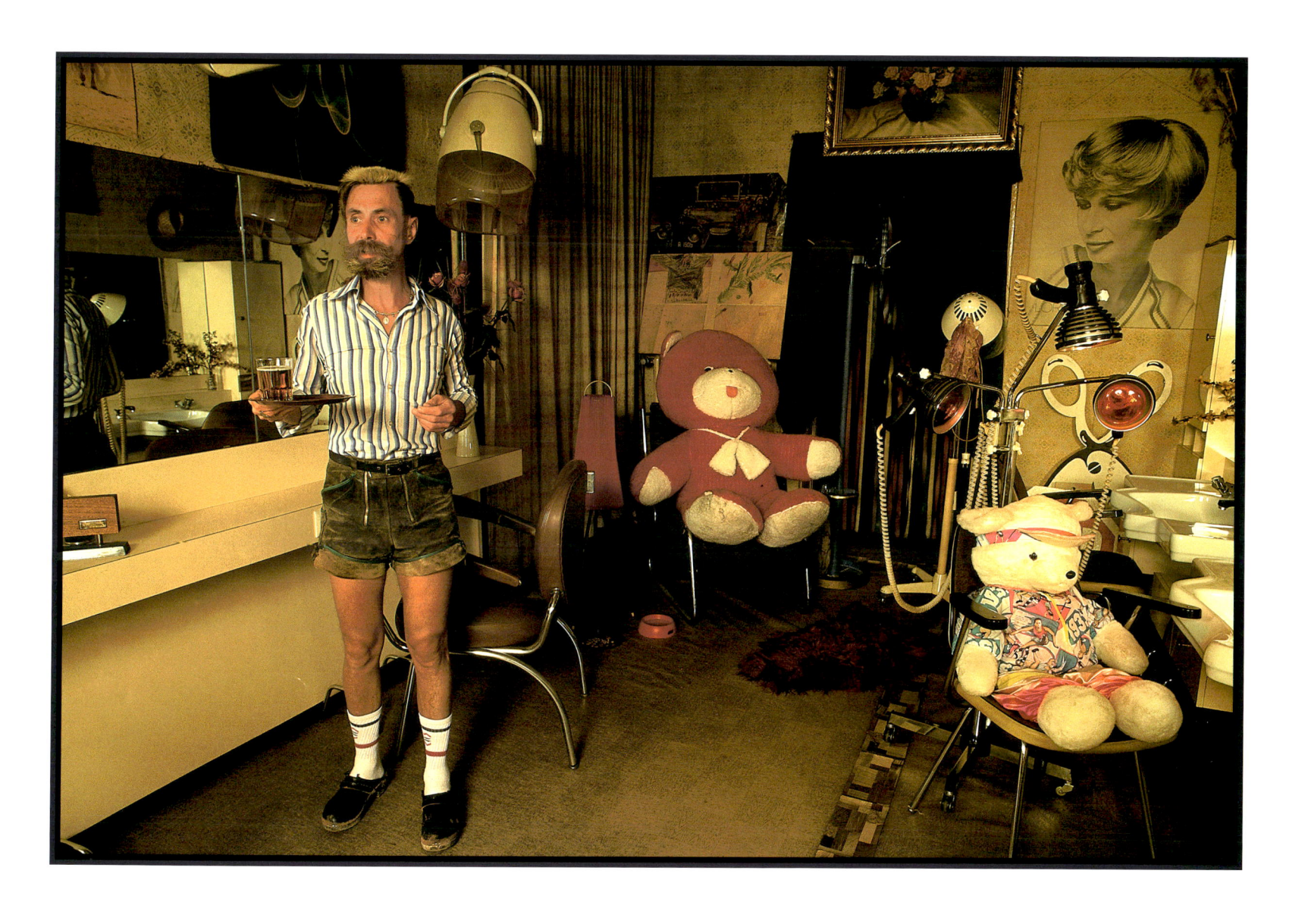

"ALFONS-HAIR-DISCO-SHOP" in Berlin's Lützowstrasse is just as individualistic as its owner. He loves lederhosen, teddy bears, and only serves beer to his customers.

GÜNTHER TWEITMANN from Kassel delights ladies of the elder generations with his hair-art. Carefully curled and permed, they feel quite content in his hands. The hairdresser attentively listens to every trouble.

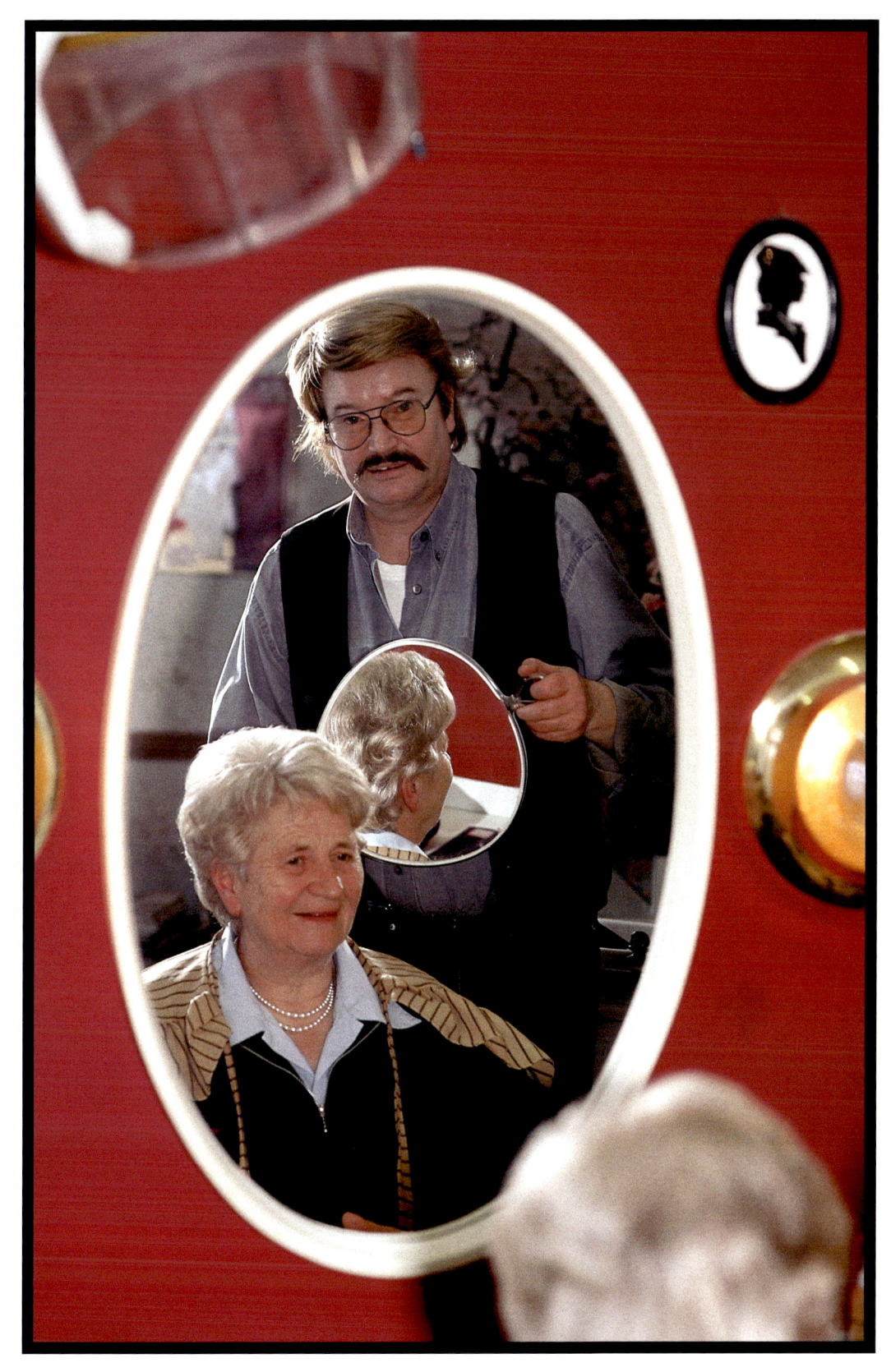

GÜNTHER TWEITMANN/KASSEL

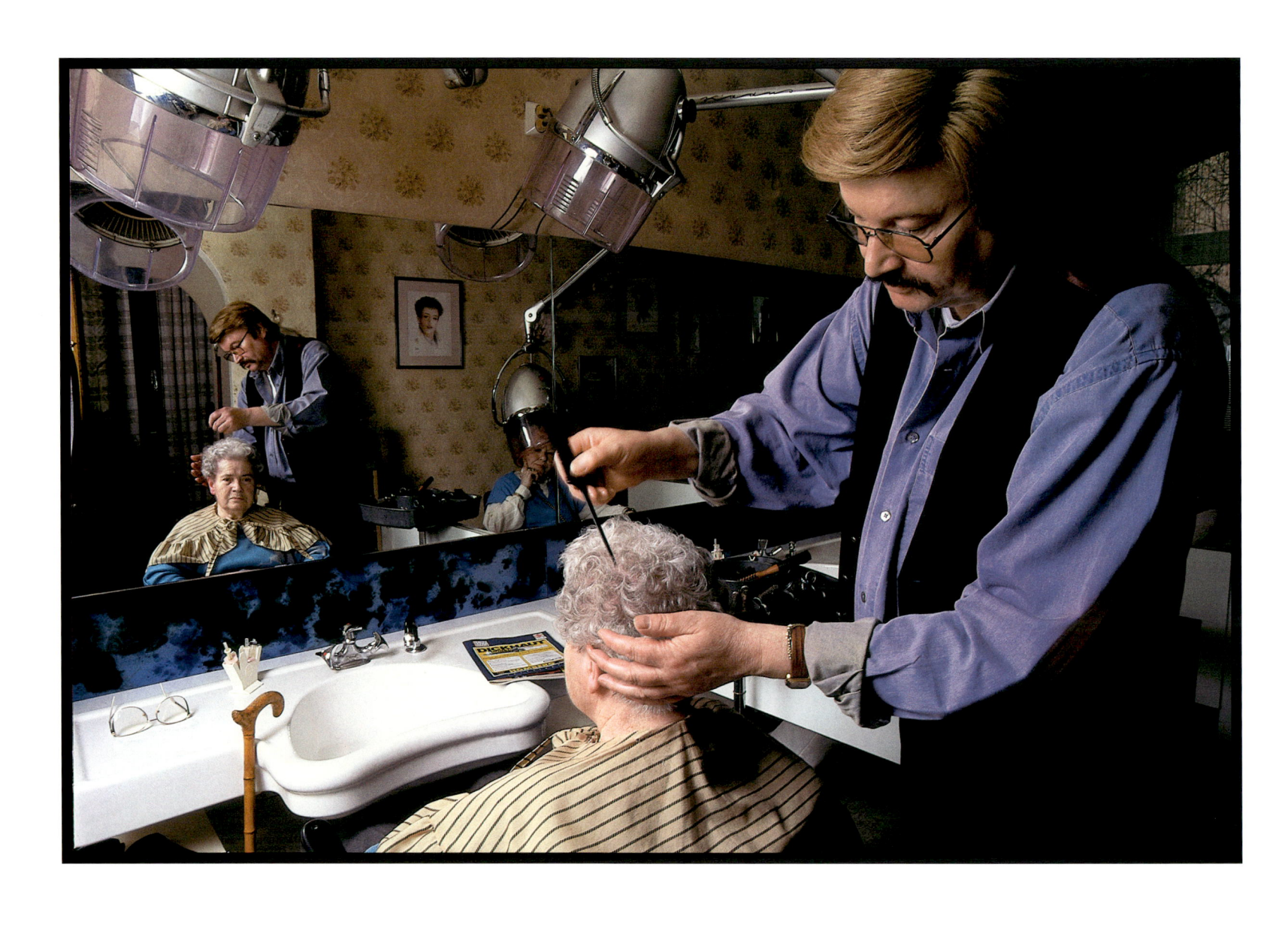

71

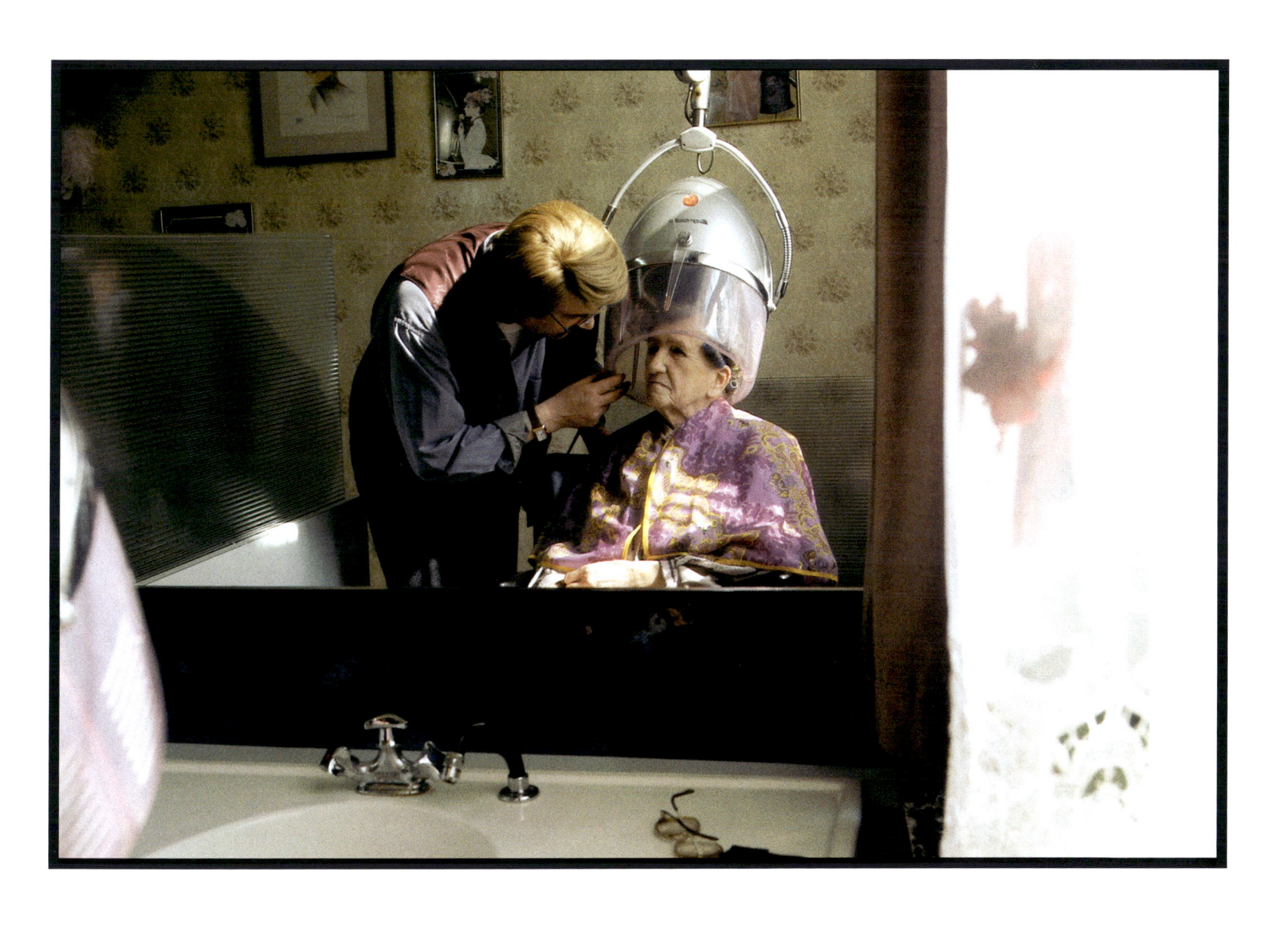

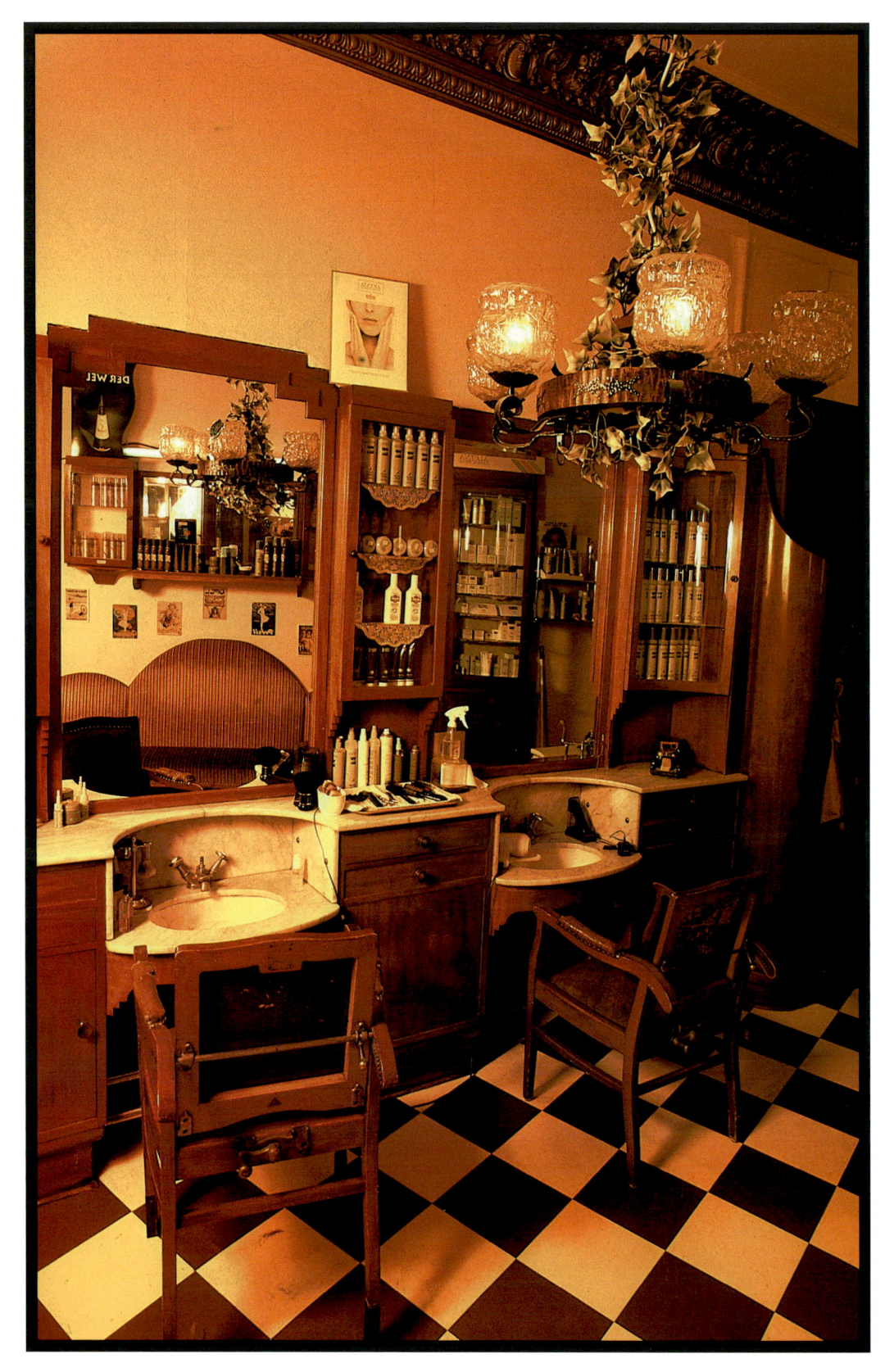

SALON OSMANI/HAMBURG

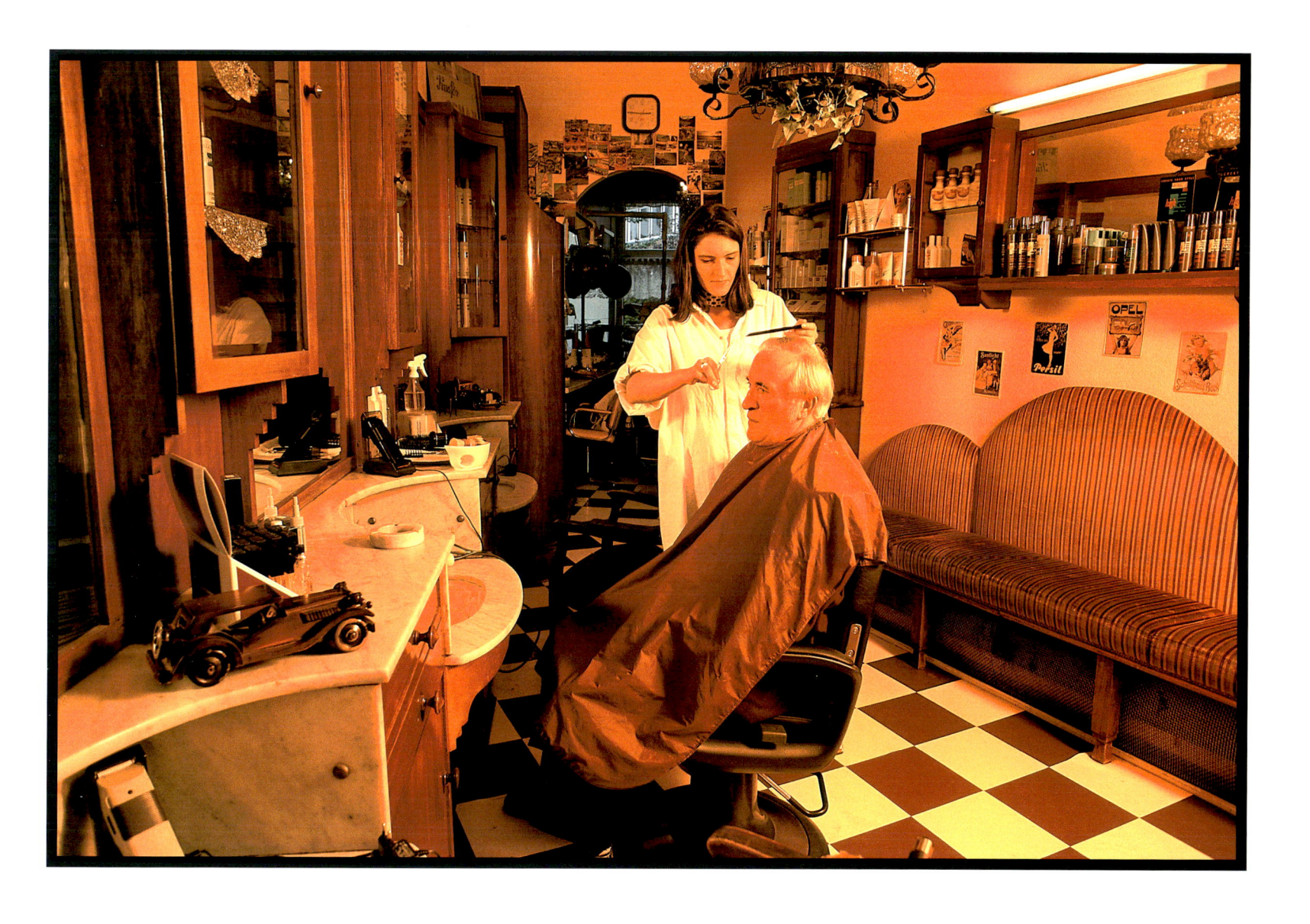

A RARE JEWEL: The hair-salon at the Hamburg Grossneumarkt, with its completely preserved interior from the 1920's. Chairs and marble sinks have survived the modernization-mania of the economic miracle. His tradition-minded customers from the neighborhood are grateful.

The born Ukrainian loves the soccer team "Frankfurt Eintracht," images of the Virgin Mary, and antique bric-a-brac. The soccer fan has lovingly adorned his Frankfurt salon altar-like with all his devotional articles.

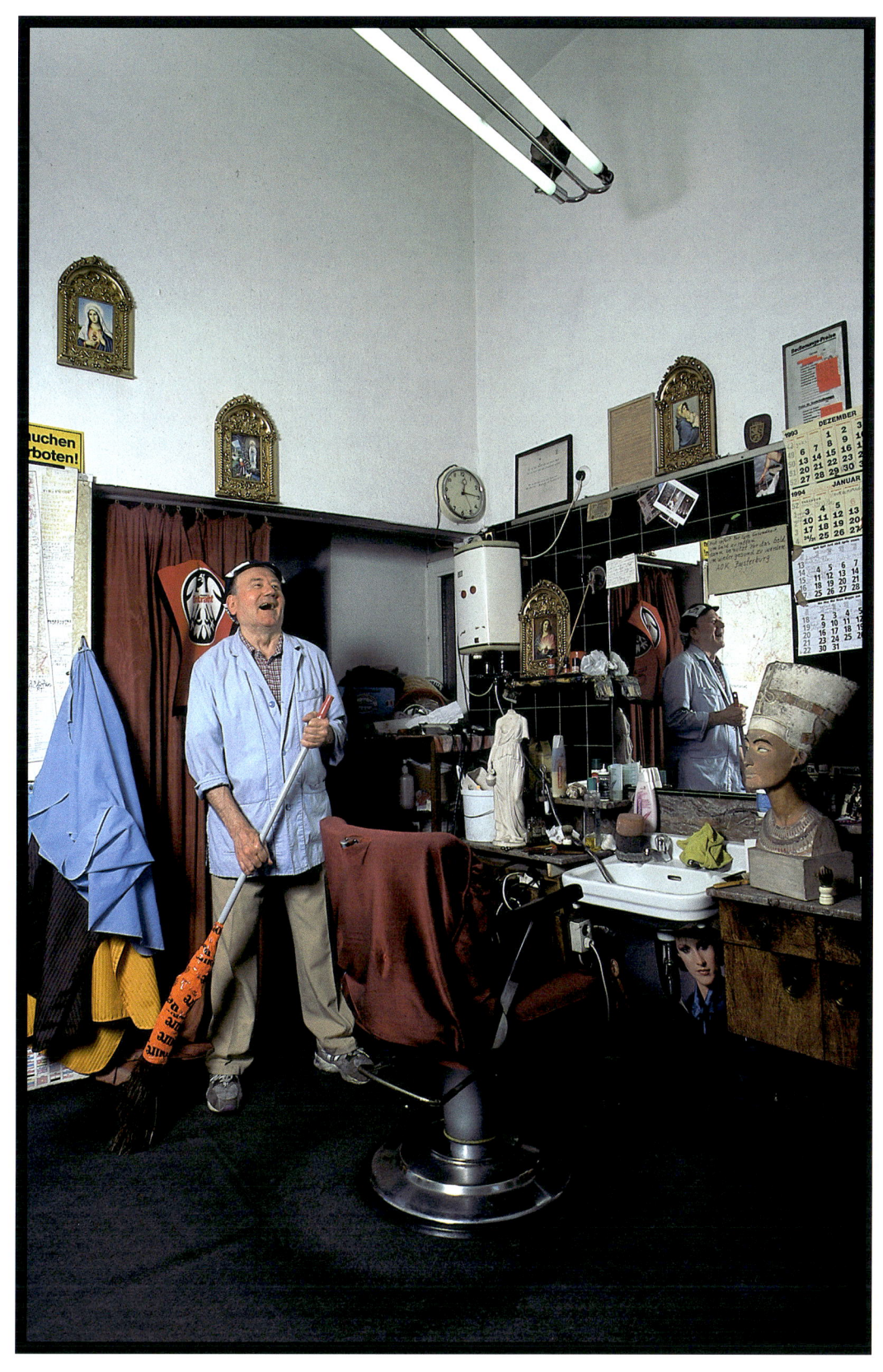

SALON SAWCZUK/FRANKFURT

Hairy Times

A Journey through Metropolis

WHETHER GIANT new constructions, decaying old buildings, sinful bars or idyllic parks: Berlin's image is as extreme and manifold as the creations of its hair-artists Horst Chudy, Markus Krause, and Frank Schäfer. Extravagantly-shrill, tragically-theatrical, noble and unique is their art. Their presentations take place at known Berlin locations: a hair-raising journey through the Spree Metropolis.

Frank Schäfer

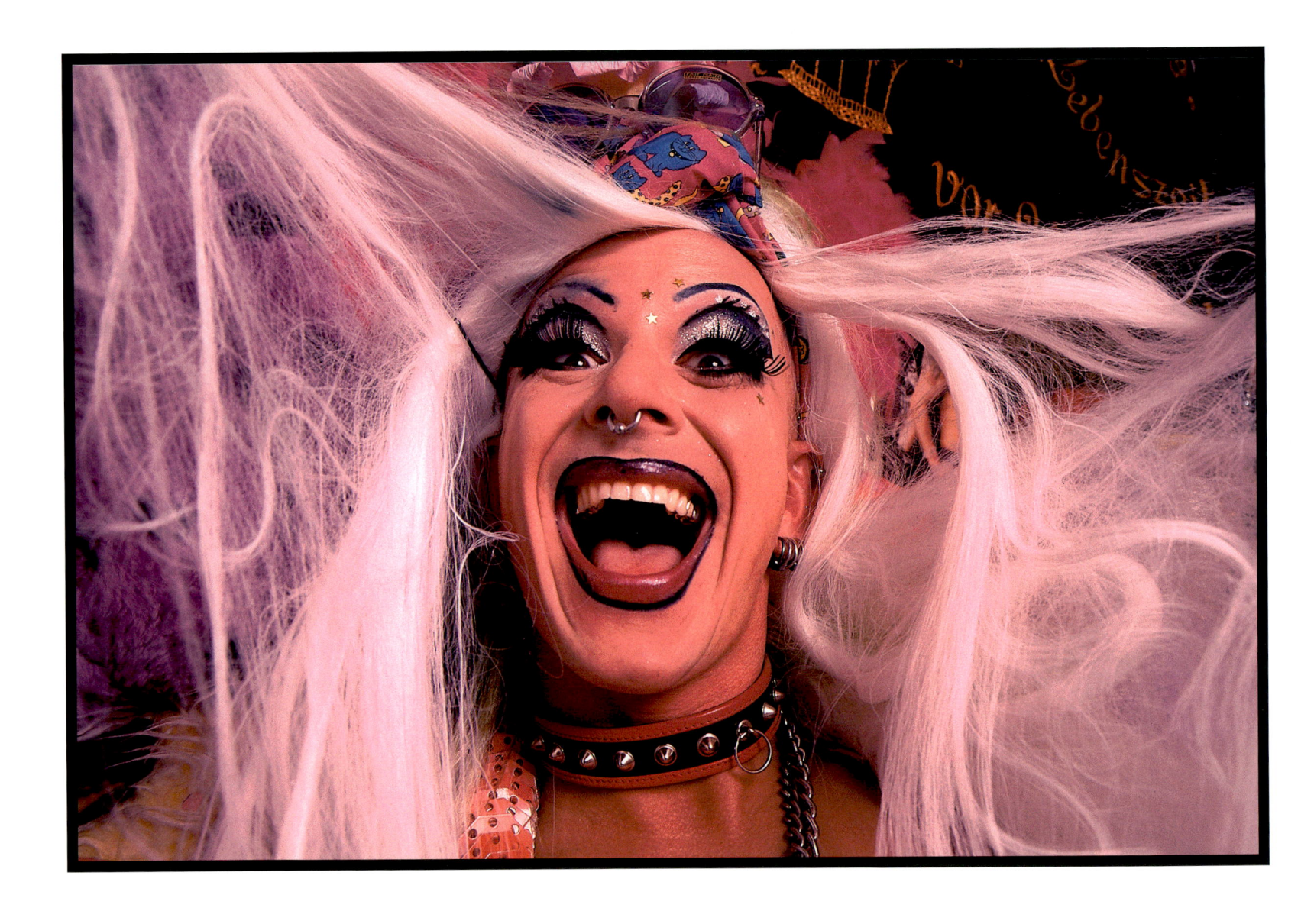

FRANK SCHÄFER, avowed gay, loves camouflage. As a child, the son of a renowned GDR-actor got a kick out of dressing up. In the former nation of workers and peasants, Schäfer's uniqueness stood out before the Prenzlauer Berg's scene was ever "in."

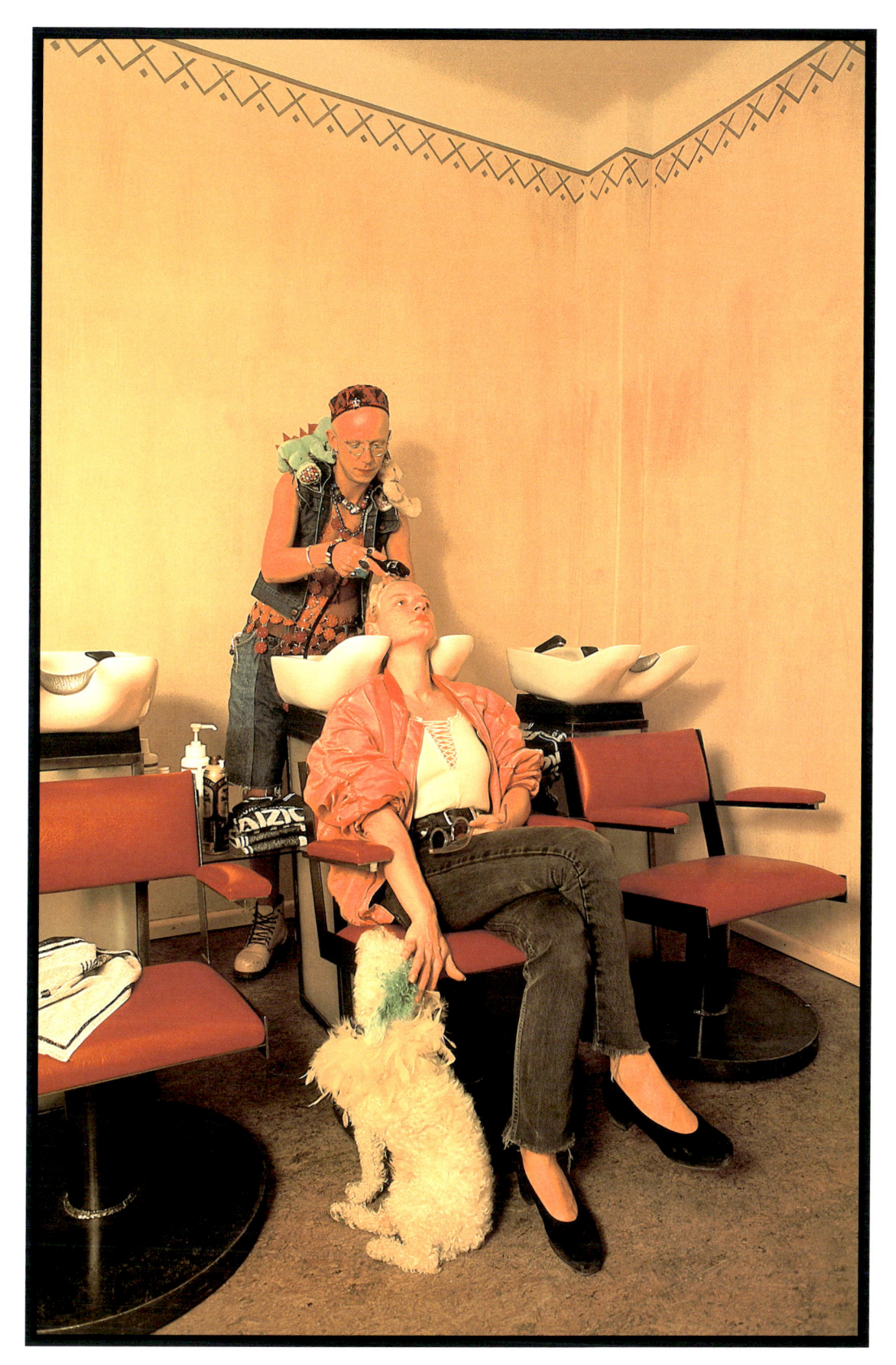

FRANK SCHÄFER has been working as a hairdresser since 1978. He broke off his studies in make-up and fashion design. But even in the old GDR days, he attracted attention with his flippy fashion shows and was active in the movie industry. His customers love his self-irony and his visual instinct. He loves his poodle "Flöckchen" and colors his hair, too.

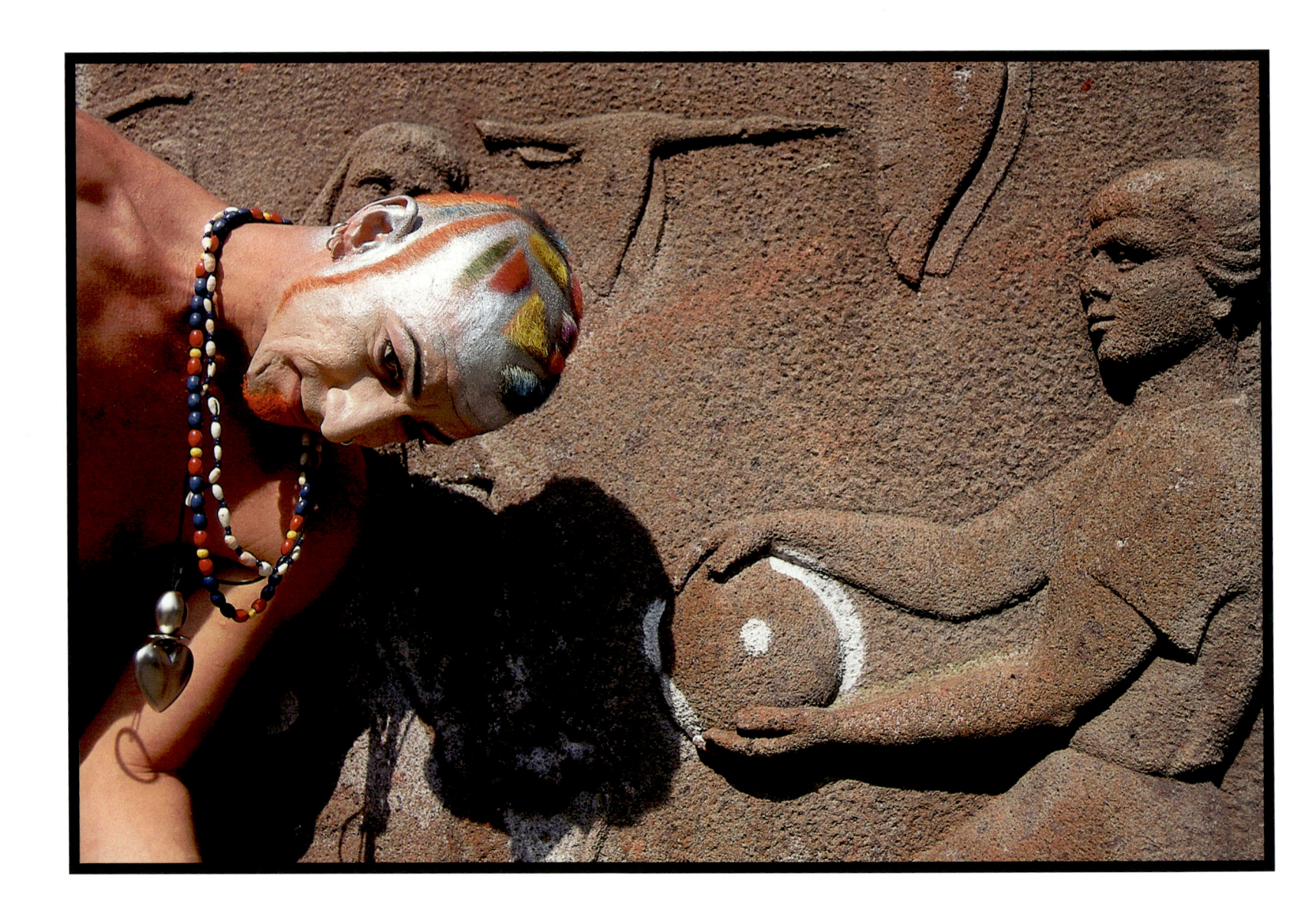

WILD AND COLORFUL: Frank Schäfer's hair-art. He has shaved and colored a mosaic onto André Jansen's head.

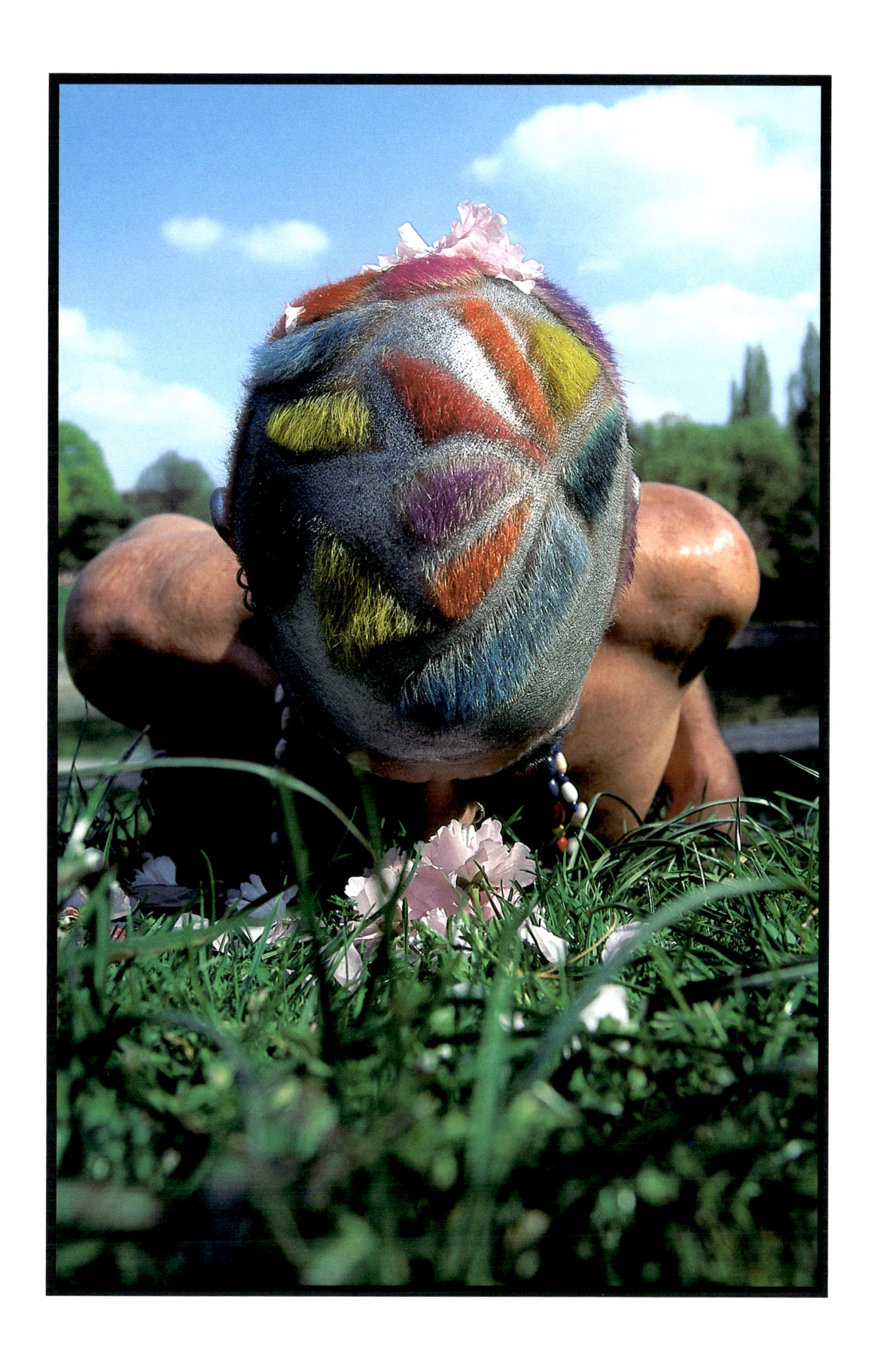

FELT PENS AND PEARLS for one's dearest spot. In the Berlin haircutting business, Frank Schäfer, inventor of intimate styling, embellishes curls in the trousers with a shave, crayons, and braided-in feathers. Young and older generations alike enjoy presenting themselves this way as a little birthday surprise.

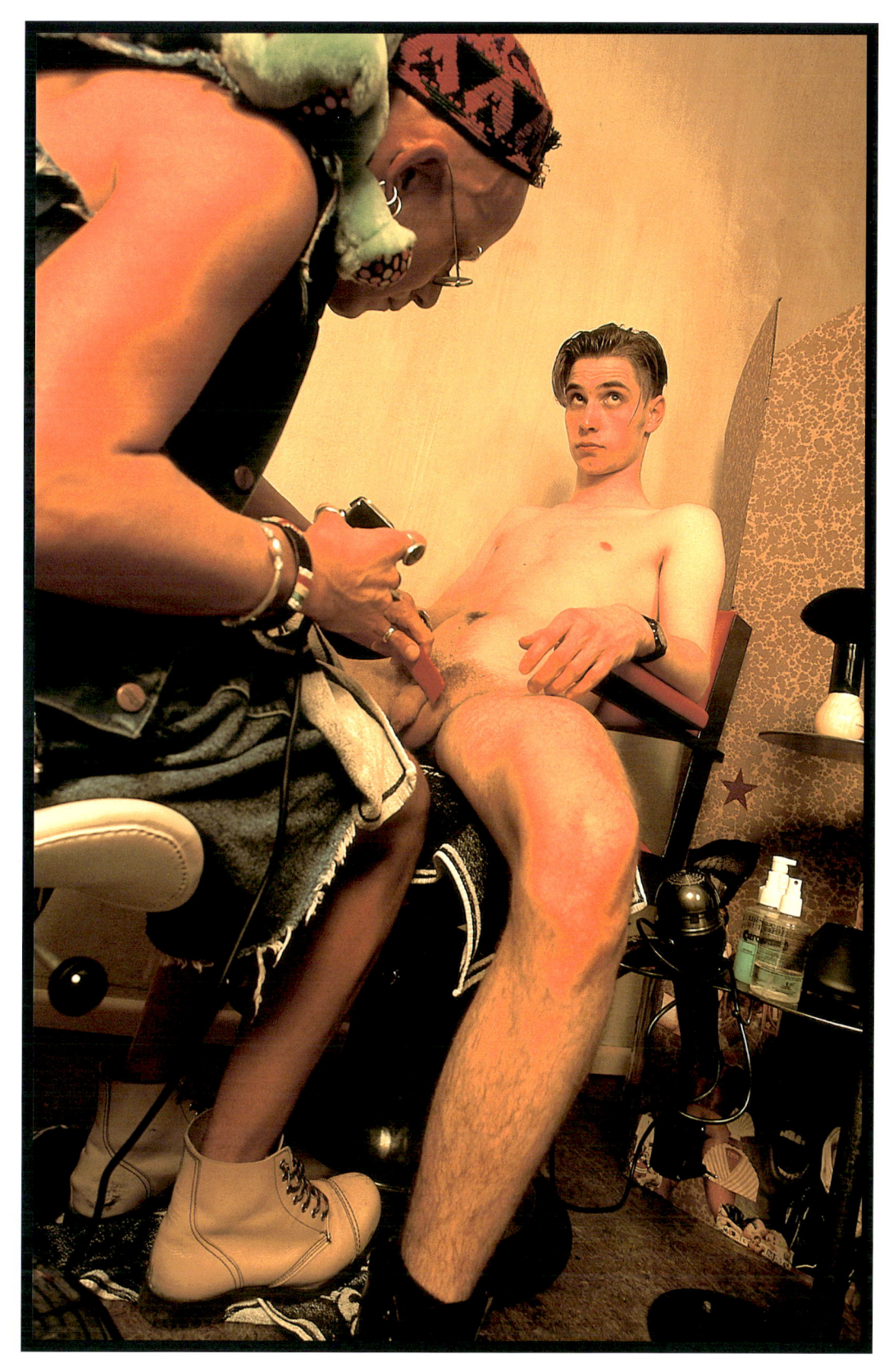

FRANK SCHÄFER/BERLIN

Horst Chudy/Markus Krause

IN THE FASHIONABLE club "Roses" in Oranienstrasse, Horst Chudy sprays the last touch onto Dagmar's do "Petite Fleur". He and Markus Krause are renowned for their show "Hair Times" at the Berlin Musical-Theater.

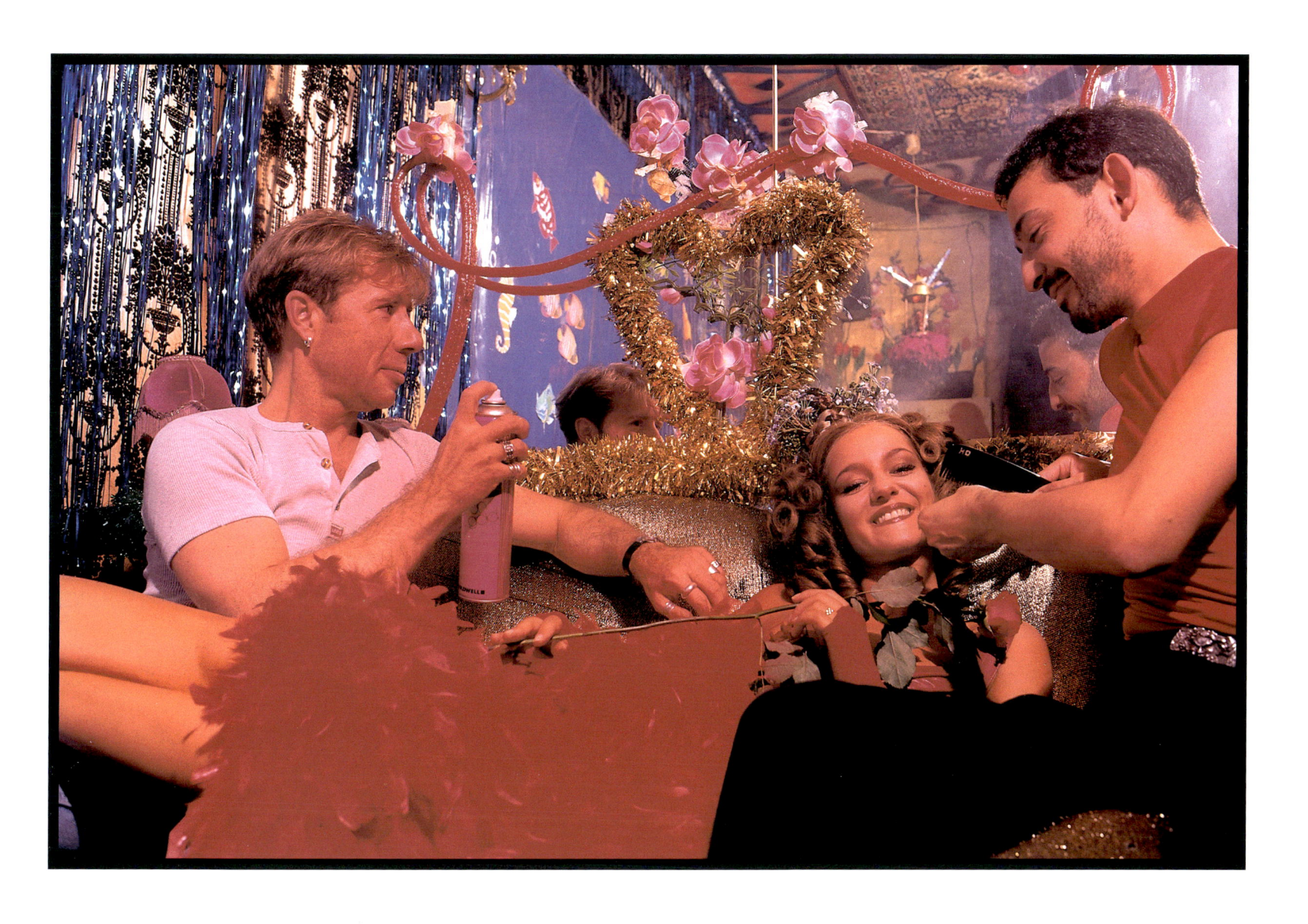

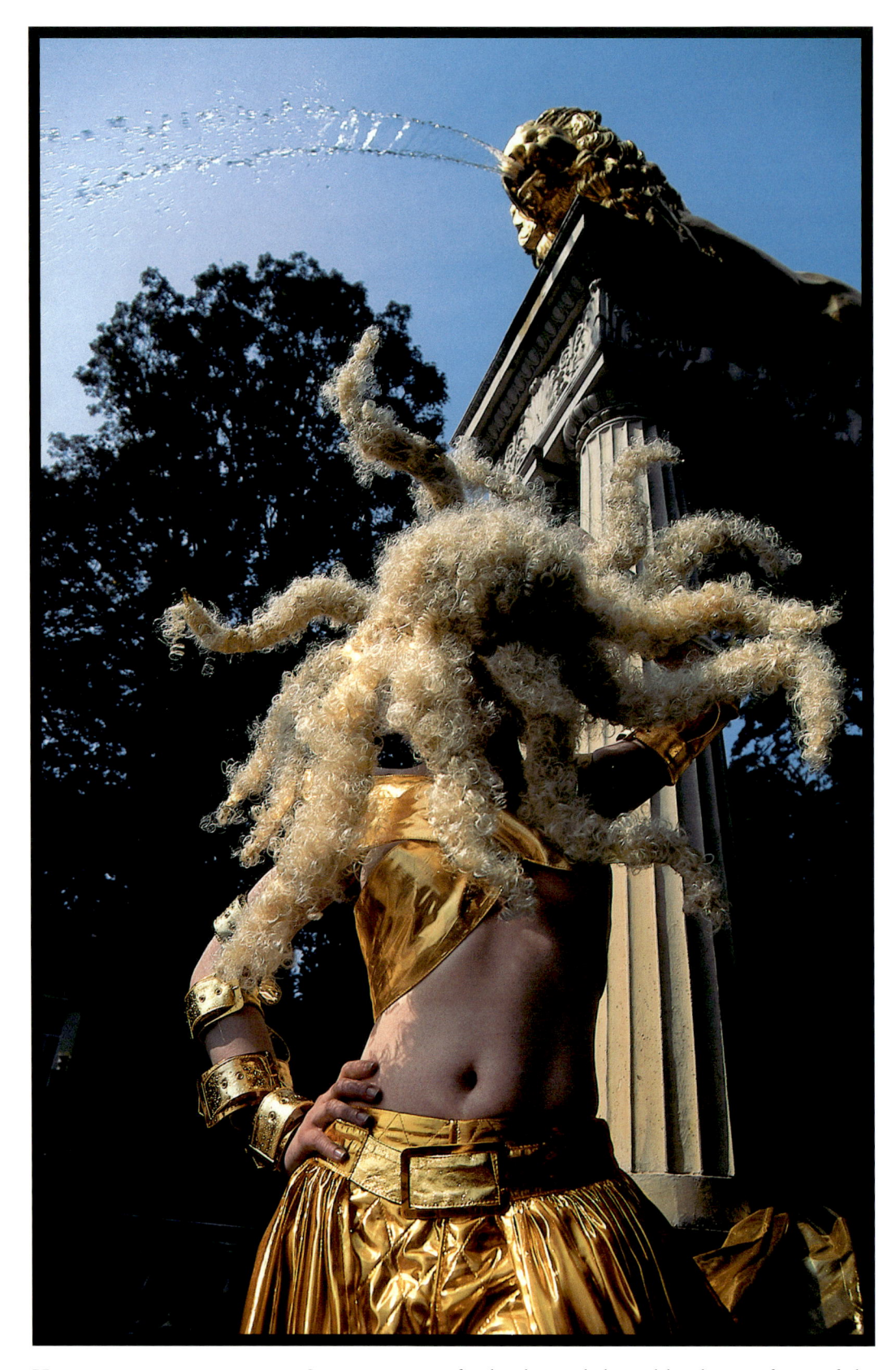

HERE COMES THE SUN! Simone, image of splendor and the golden lion in front of the classicistic "Schloss Glienicke," both with bright manes.

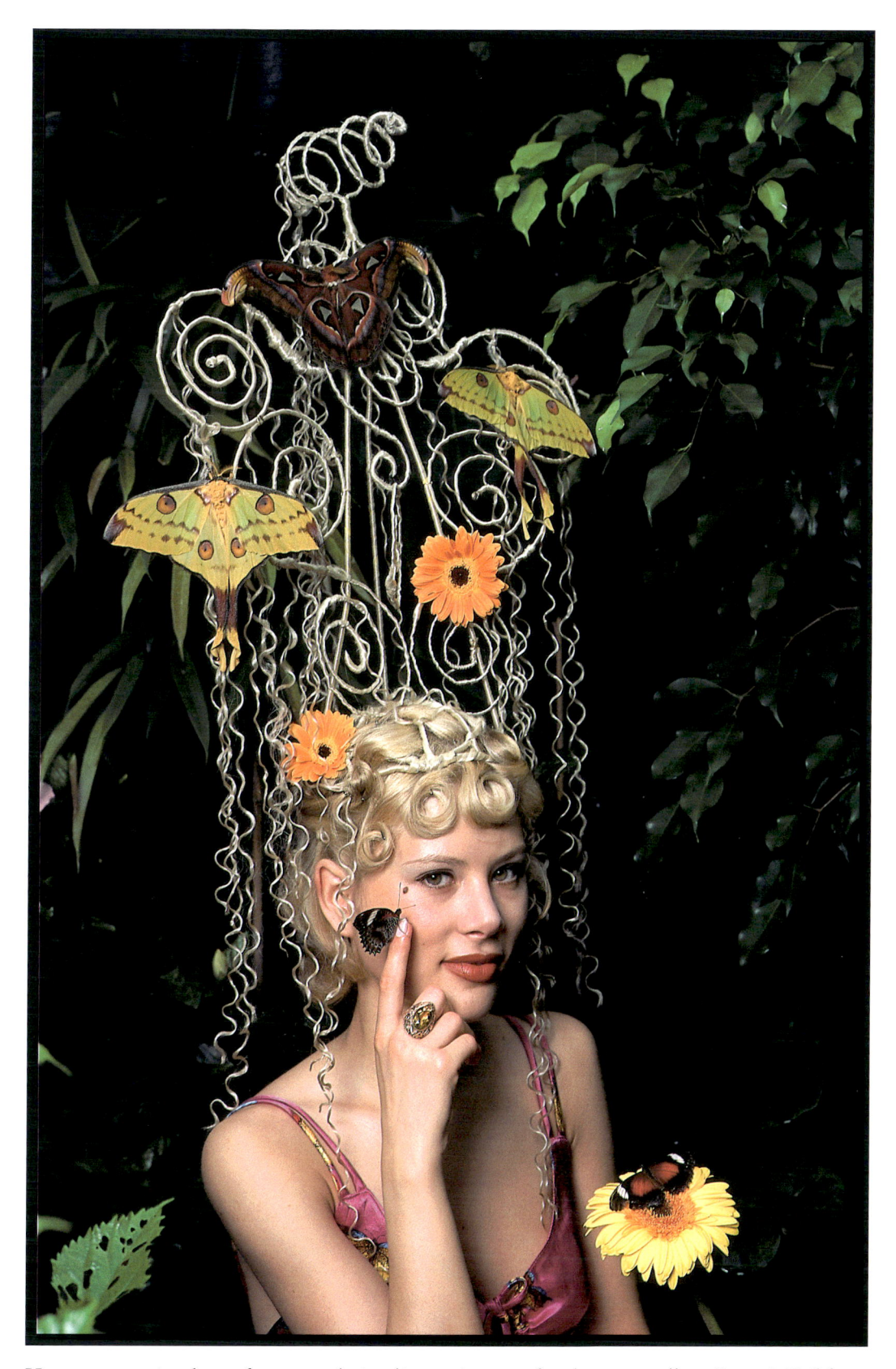

HAIRSPRAY in place of nectar: a hairy disappointment for the great yellow Comet's Tail from Madagascar and all the other exotically colorful moths at "Haus Schmetterlingslust" (House of Butterflies) at the Britzer Garten. Maren's crown of wire, wrapped with shiny, blond hair only deceives the drowsy butterflies for a short time. Then they fly on.

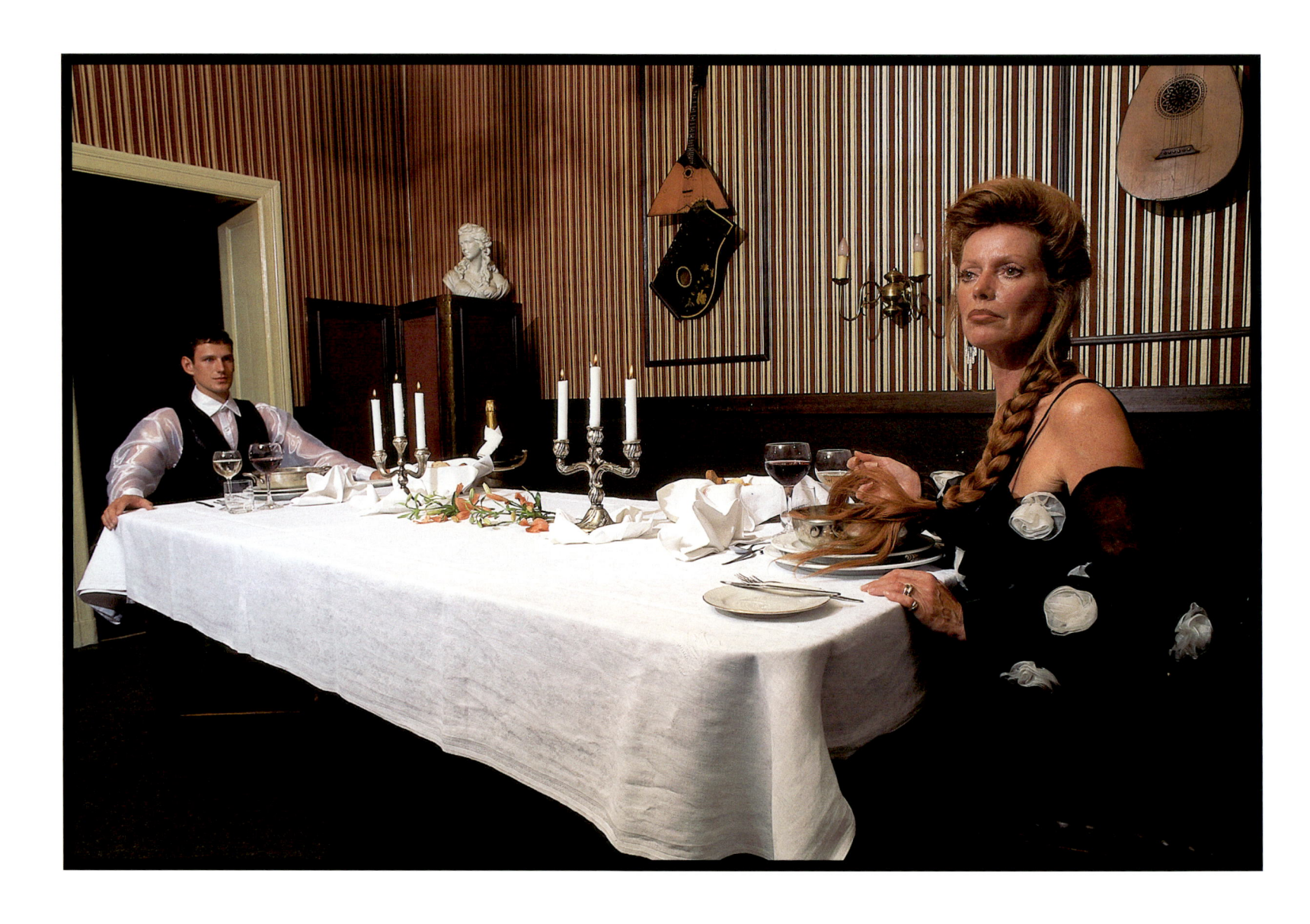

NOT ONLY hair in the soup: in the "Offenbacher Stuben" at Prenzlauer Berg Irene discovers her entire braid in her soup bowl.

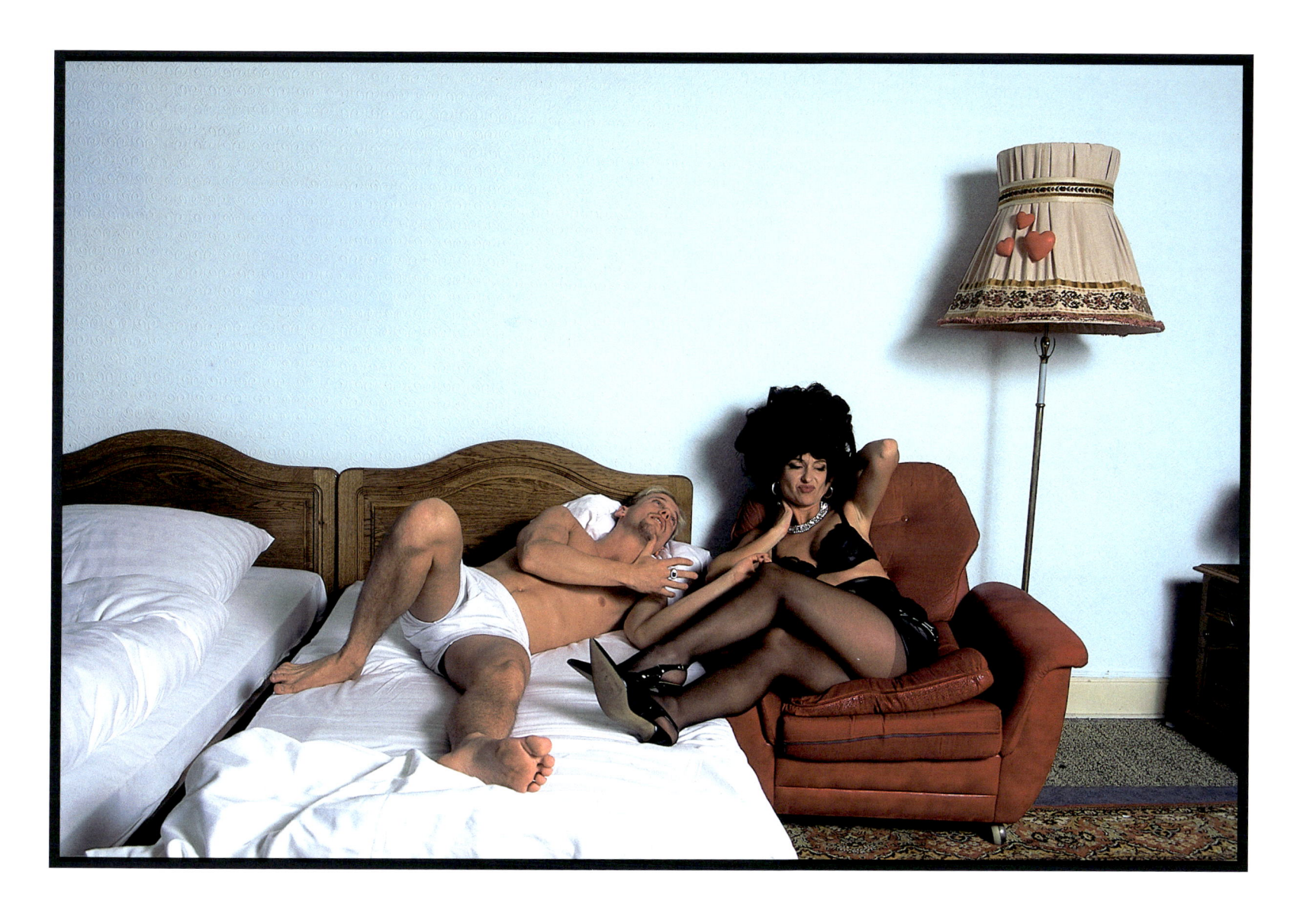

"DARLING MY HAIR!" The heavy "Farah Diva" hair-do in the style of the sixties keeps men at bay. Madame prefers sleeping in the red vinyl armchair of "Hotel Insel Rügen" in the Pariser Strasse.

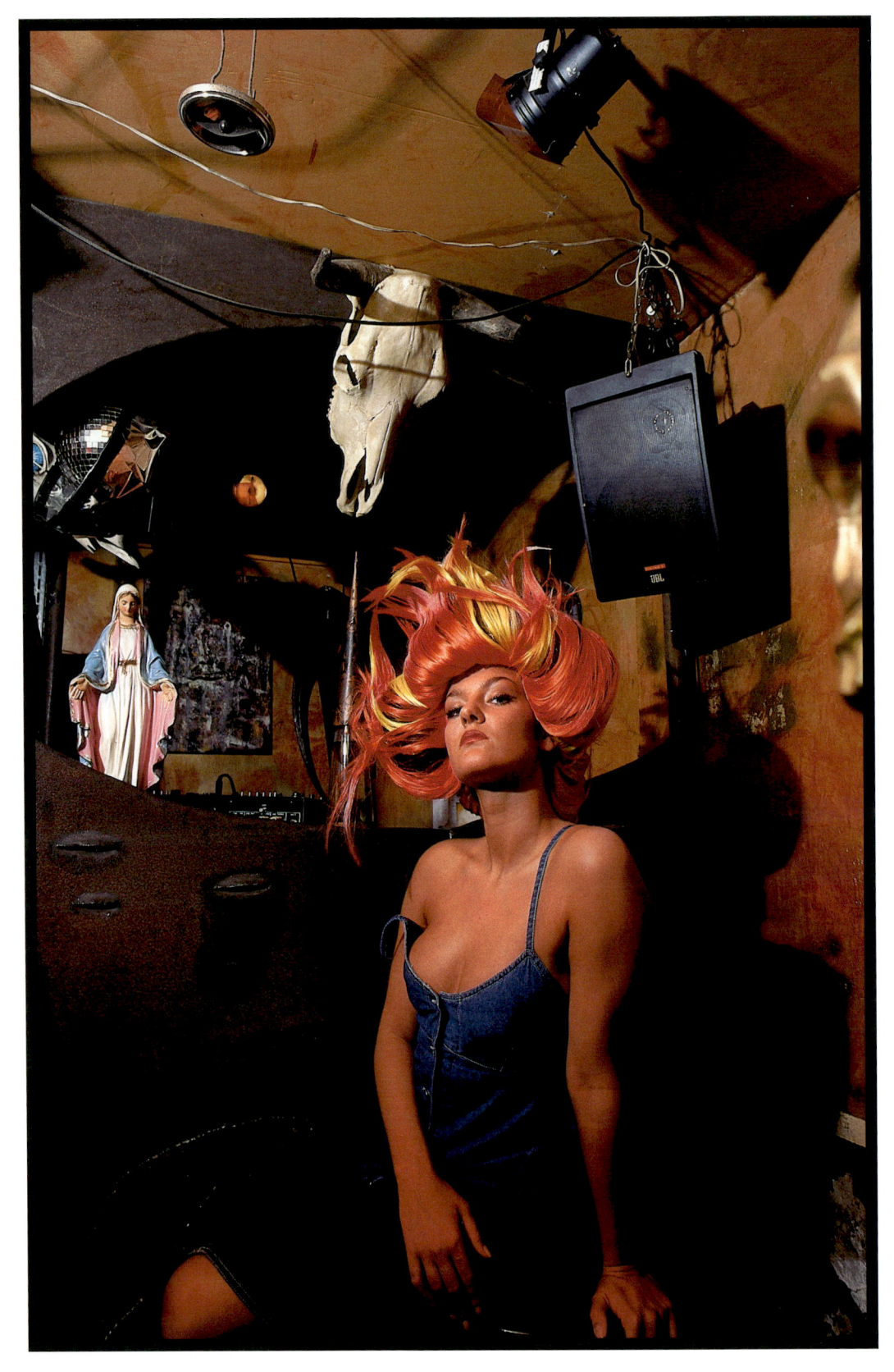

"FIRE AND FLAME" for long nights with a blazing mop of hair. Horst Chudy helped nature along with elaborate color-effects.

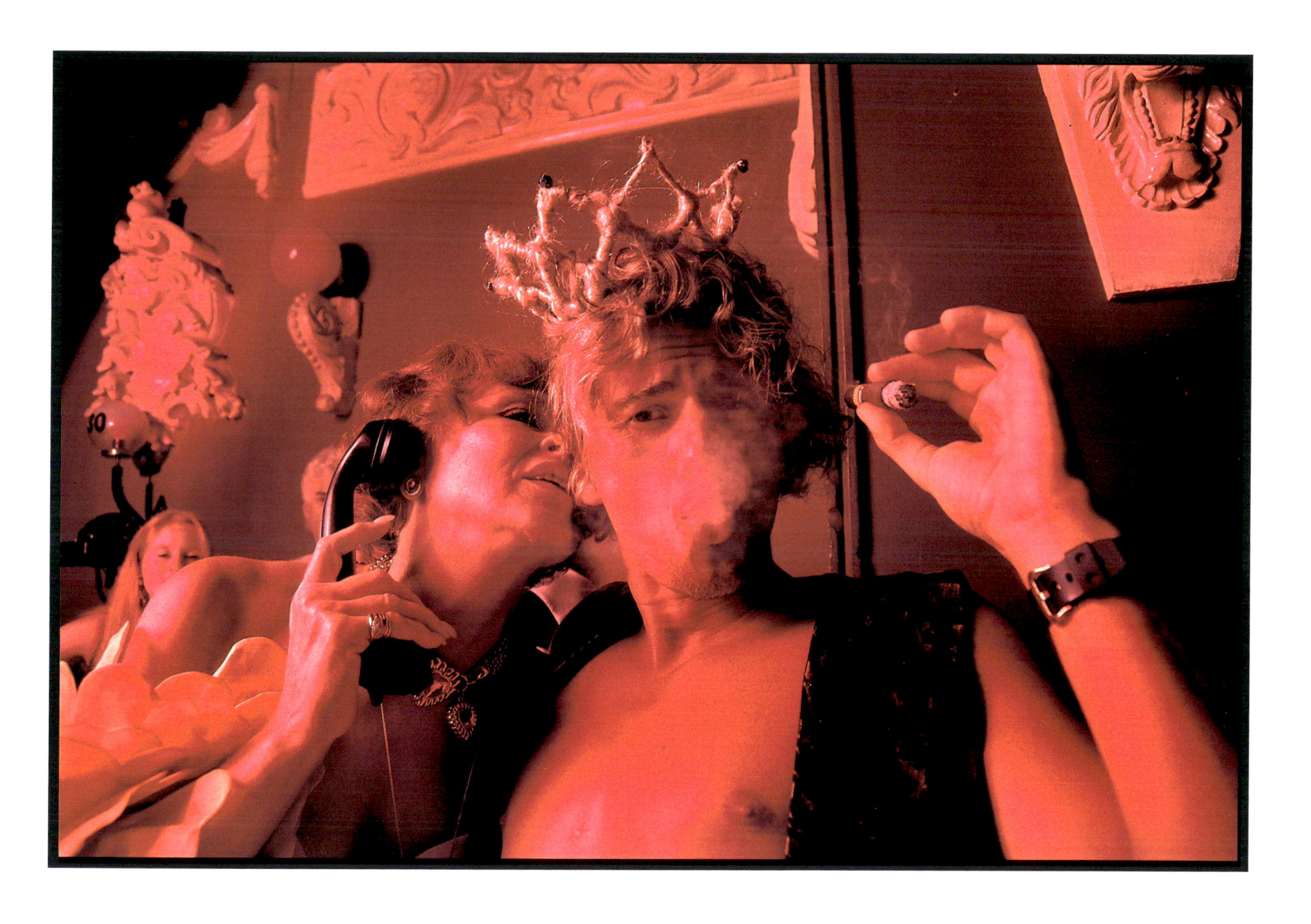

"CROWN OF LIFE": at Ballhaus Berlin, a dancing establishment in the Chausseestrasse, meeting point for lonely hearts and the elder generation, anyone can find her fairy-tale prince. Sometimes he will even be wearing a crown with real hair twisted about it.

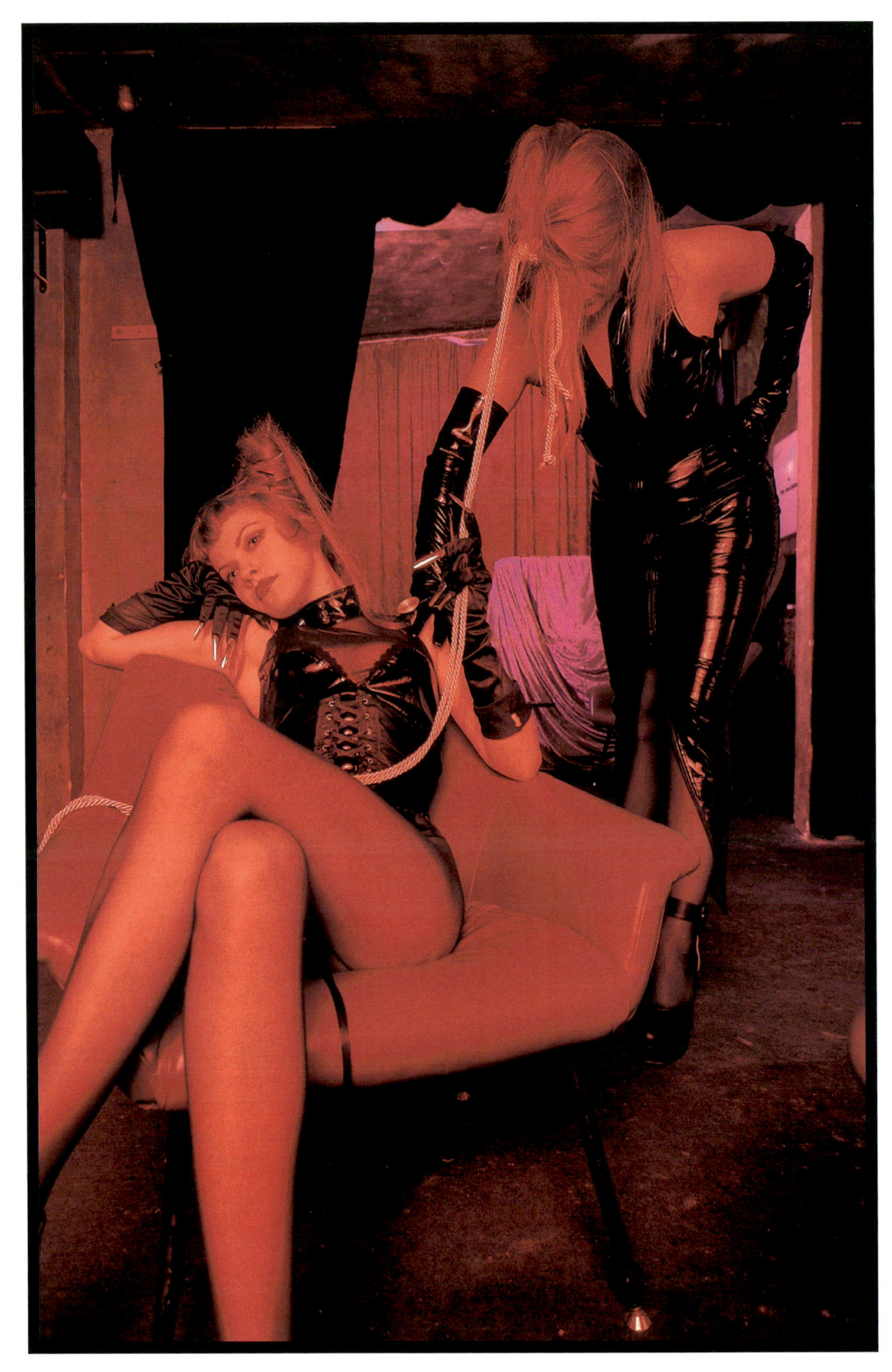

"GETTING IN ONE'S HAIR". From torture of love to sweet pain, the lust of pain and hair are the story of the SM Torture-Club of "Ex-Kreuz-Club," located in a bunker in Albrechtstrasse. Here those inclined to such fetishes meet. The Ten Commandments with their own interpretations are on the wall: "You shall not steal your neighbor's possessions."

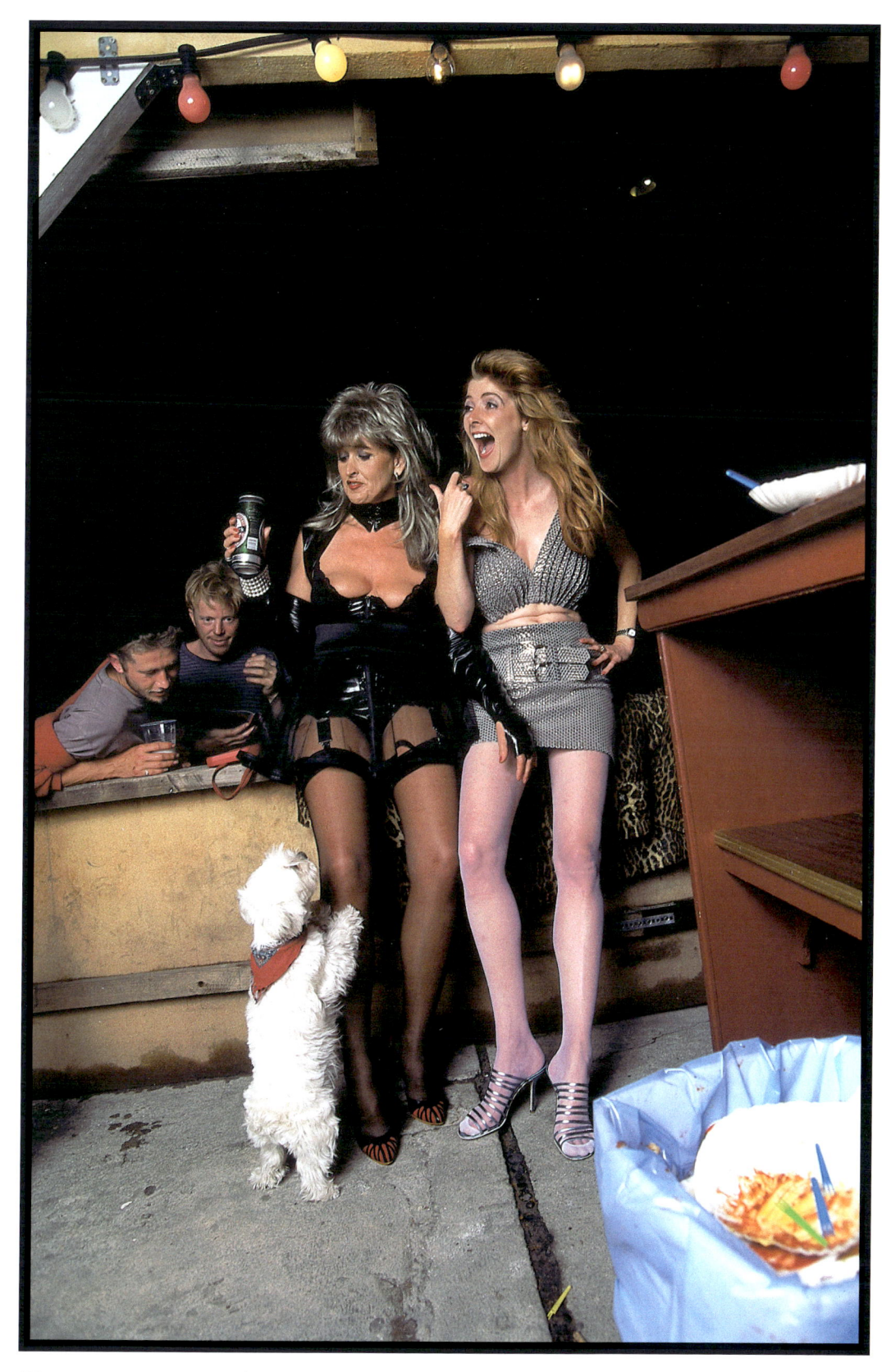

"FALSE BLONDS," a fast-food place in the Oranienburger Strasse. In the days of antiquity, the wig served as an instrument of deception. Messaline, Roman empress and whore, wore a blond wig of genuine Germanic air on her nightly escapades through the city's brothels.

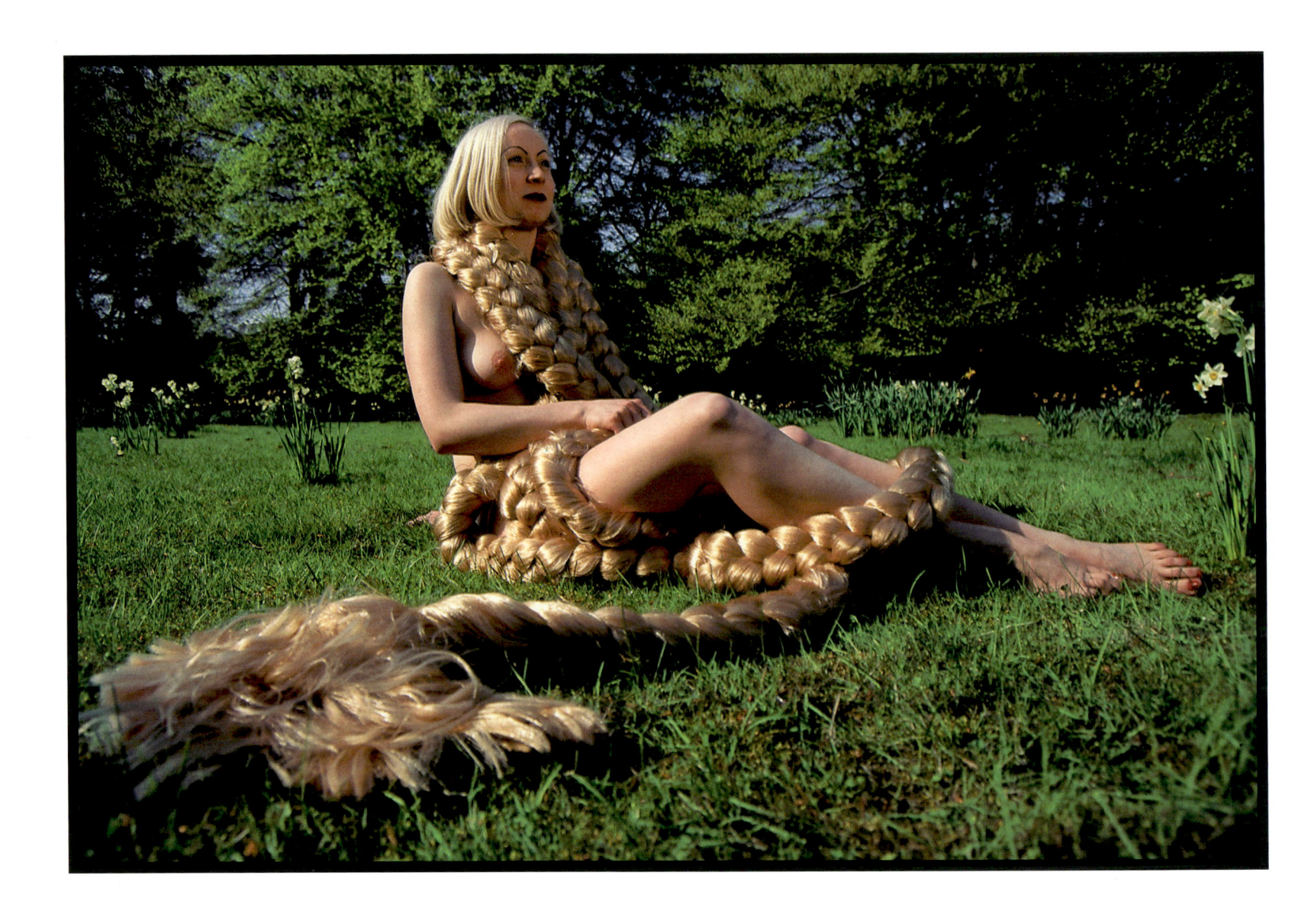

WAITING for her fairy-tale prince in a narcissus field in the Tiergarten, Rapunzel lets down her hair: she is only wearing her lengthy braid, as thick as an arm.

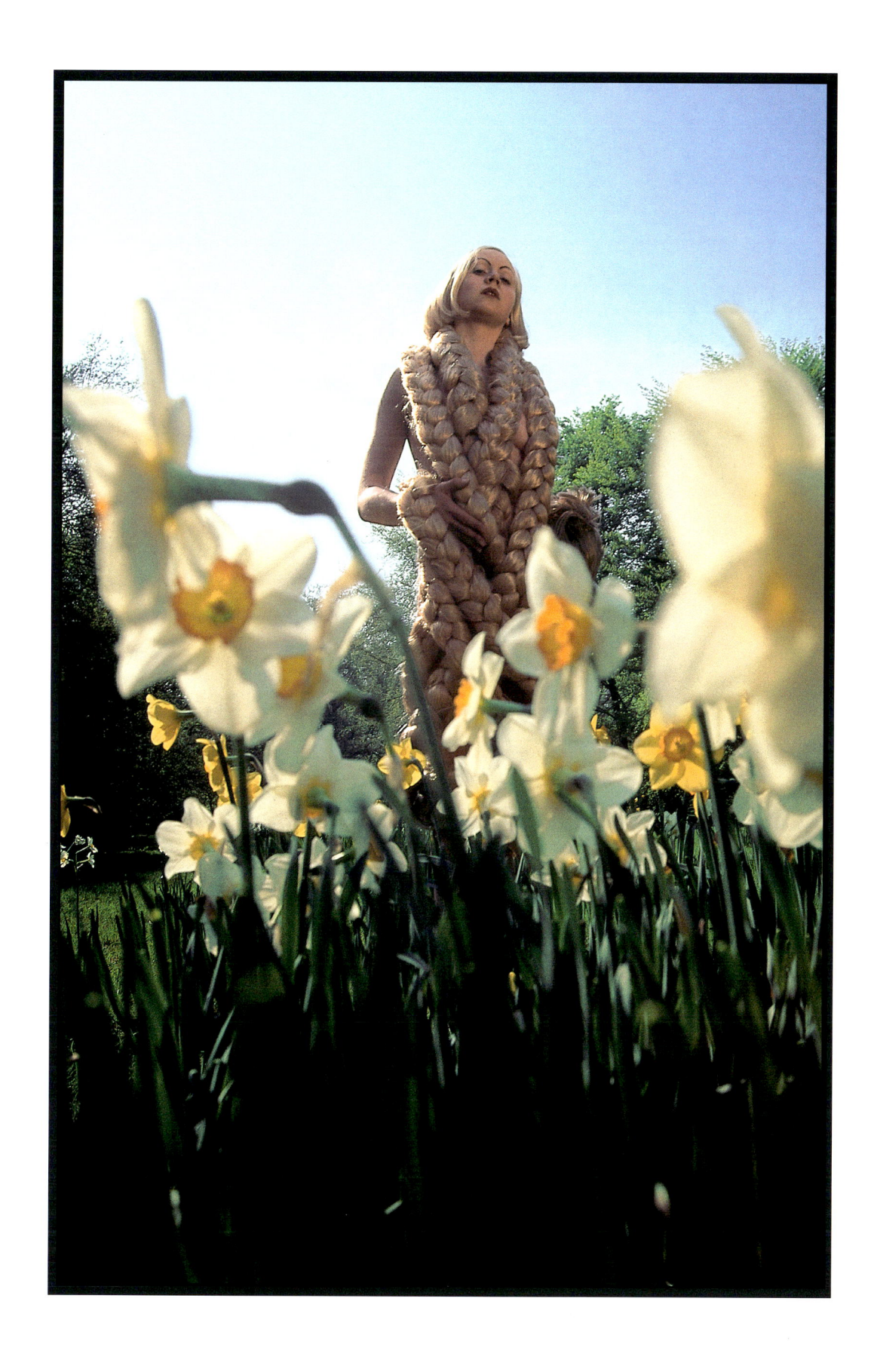

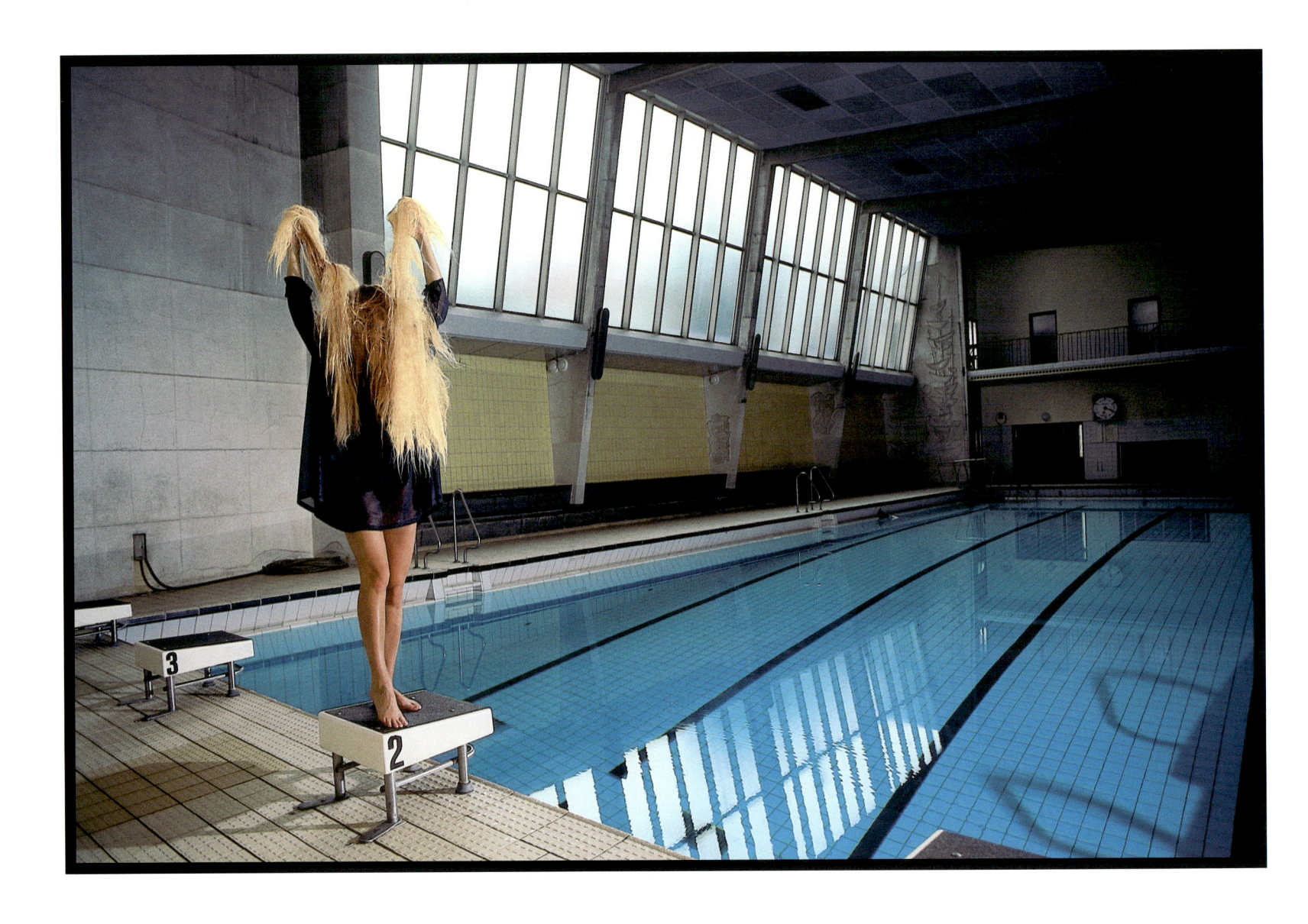

"MERMAID" with lengthy tresses, standing in "Prinzenbad," a swimming pool built in the fifties, located in Baerwaldstrasse, Berlin.

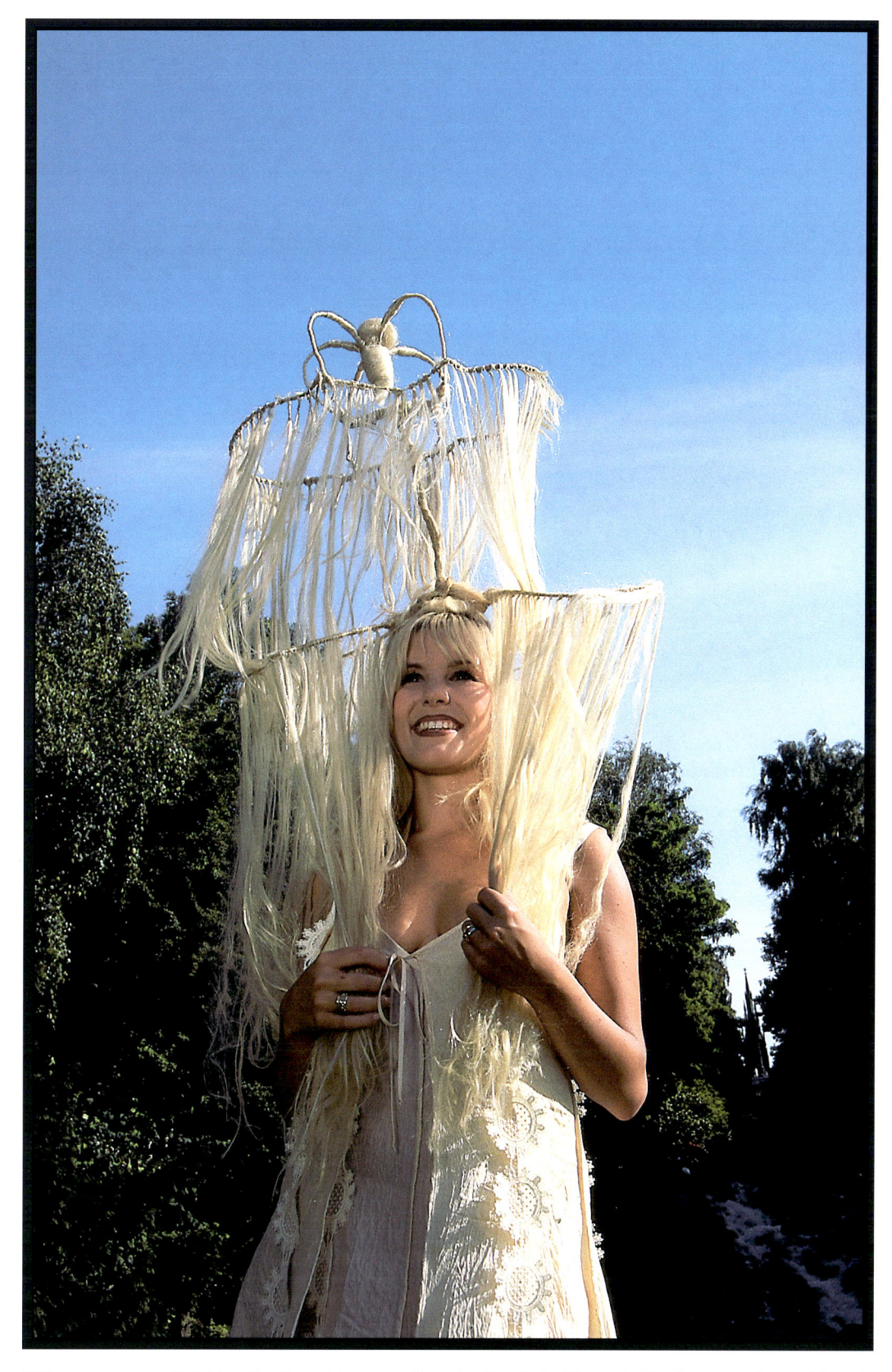

"WATERFALL": Miss Berlin 1994 standing in Berlin's Victoria Park, cascades of hand-knotted long hair flowing.

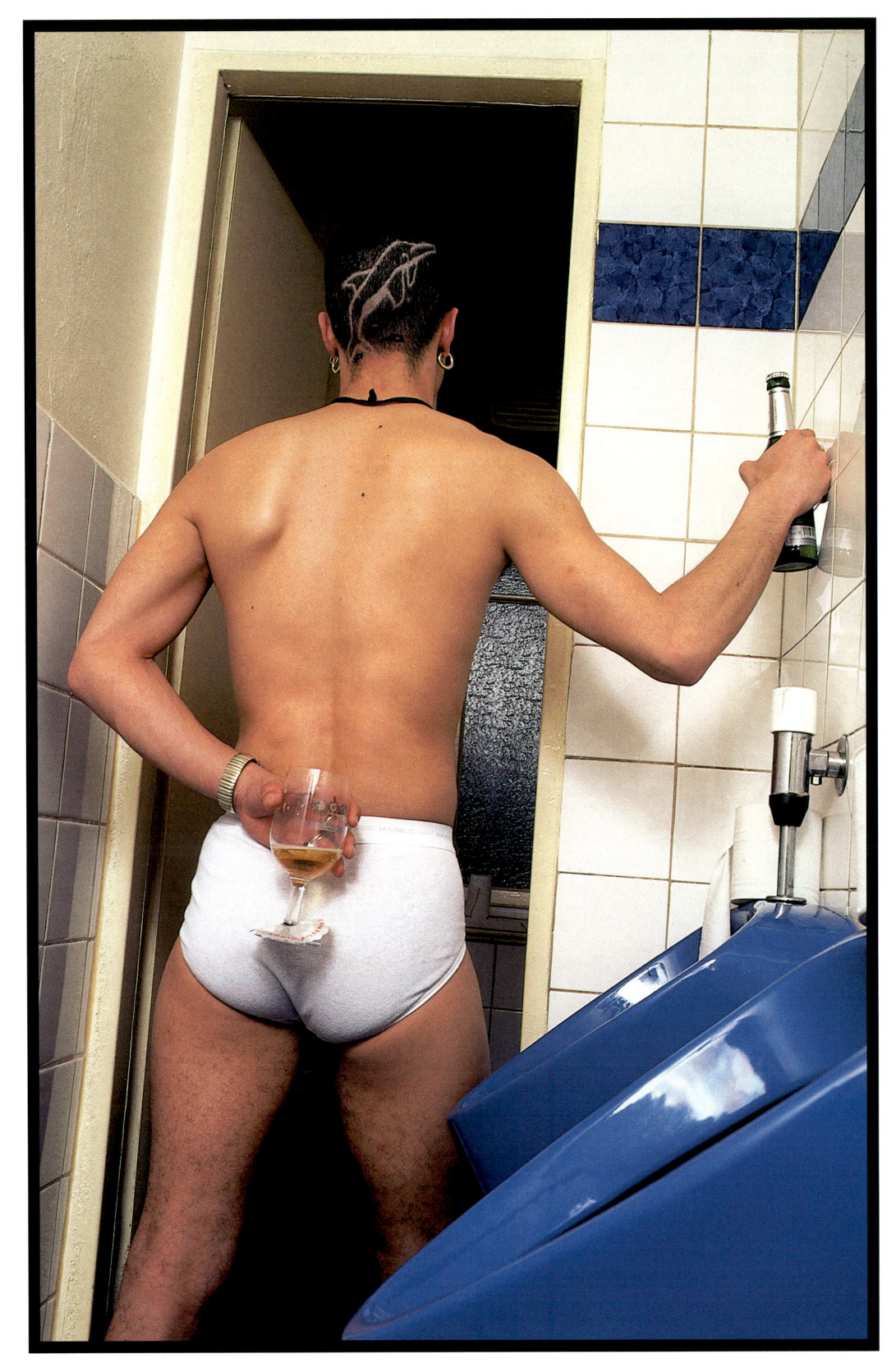

"FLIPPER." Without using a stencil, Horst Chudy shaved a dolphin onto the back of his customer's head and colored it with blue water spots.

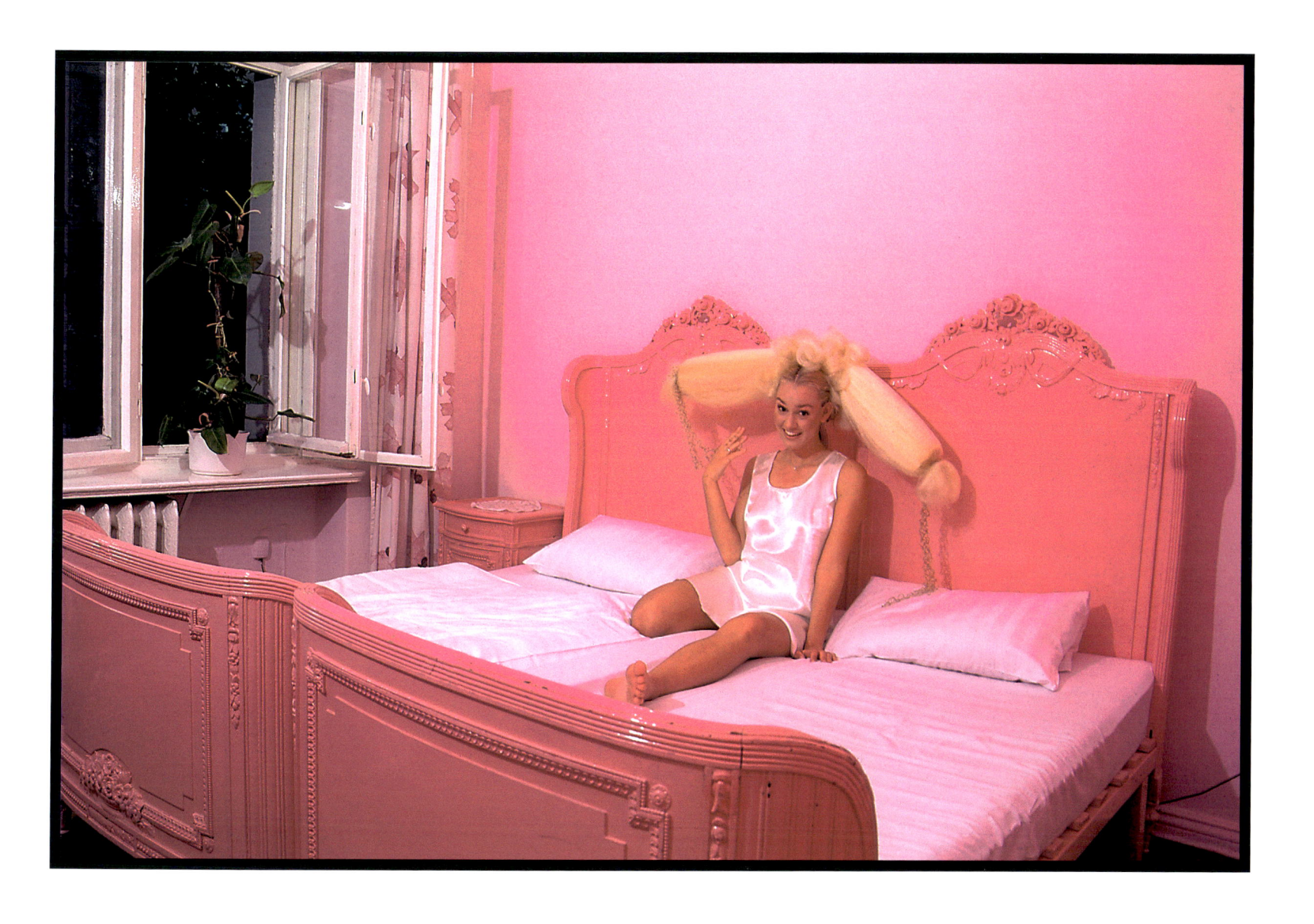

"THINK PINK." In the Biedermeier room of the Künstlerlokal Steiner (Artist's Hotel) in the Albrecht-Archilles-Strasse in Wilmersdorf, hair-art has its price: Horst Chudy's fantastic Biedermeier interpretation of bulging hair, does not exactly promise sweet dreams.

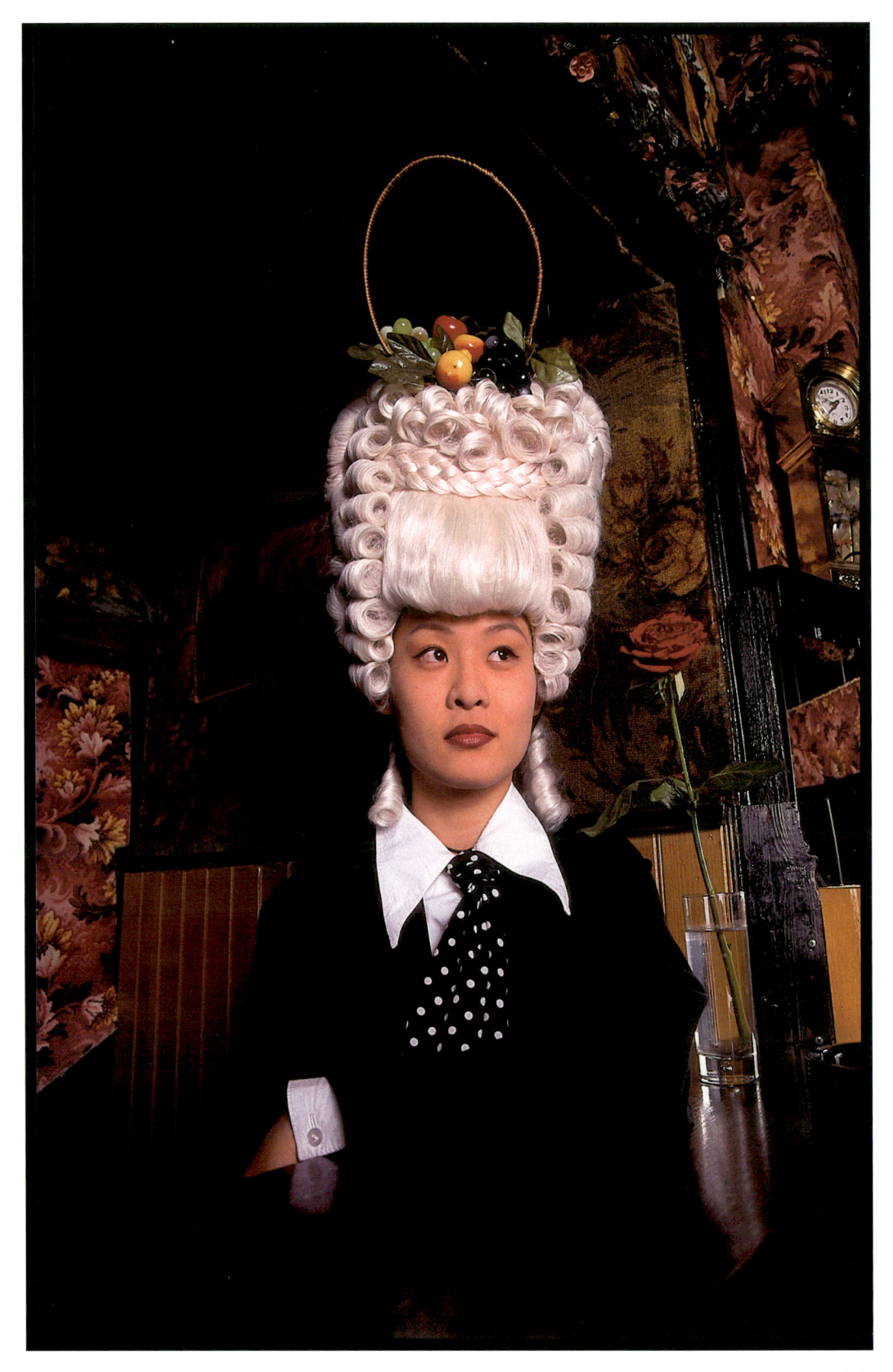

FIGAROES IN THE ERA of Louis XIV even used ladders to create the historical models for this "rococo" hairstyle. Hee Yong of Korea decorating the "Kumpelnest" in Berlin's Lützowstrasse with the coiffeur.

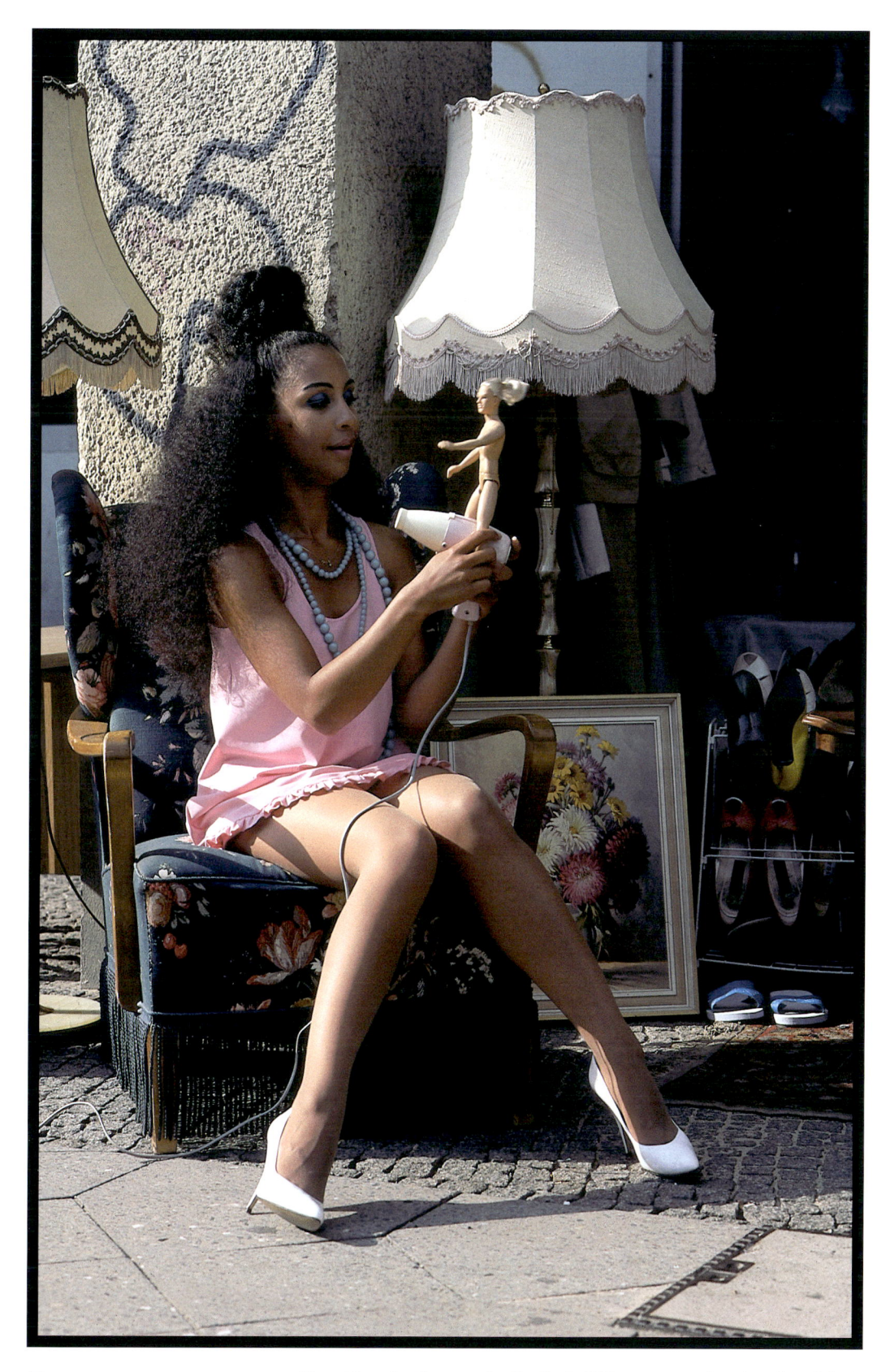

GONE WITH THE WIND. Outside a junk store in Berlin's Bülowstrasse is wig of real hair with woven-in ring of artificial hair, blown by a hair-dryer. The handy, little gadget owes its invention to two household appliances. In 1920, the warm air blower of a vacuum cleaner and the small motor of a mixer were assembled into a hair-dryer.

ANDREAS HINTZ

«Perrückt»

WIGS, not to conceal faults but to attract attention: the Hamburg make-up man and hair-artist, Andreas Hintz, creates such works in his studio "Perrückt." The artificial splendor, a work of hairy grace, is made using materials such as licorice, macaroni, foam rubber or pastry dough. Each piece is unique, and is fitted to the head by plaster cast. Thus, these special wigs fit precisely and do not require much styling.

109

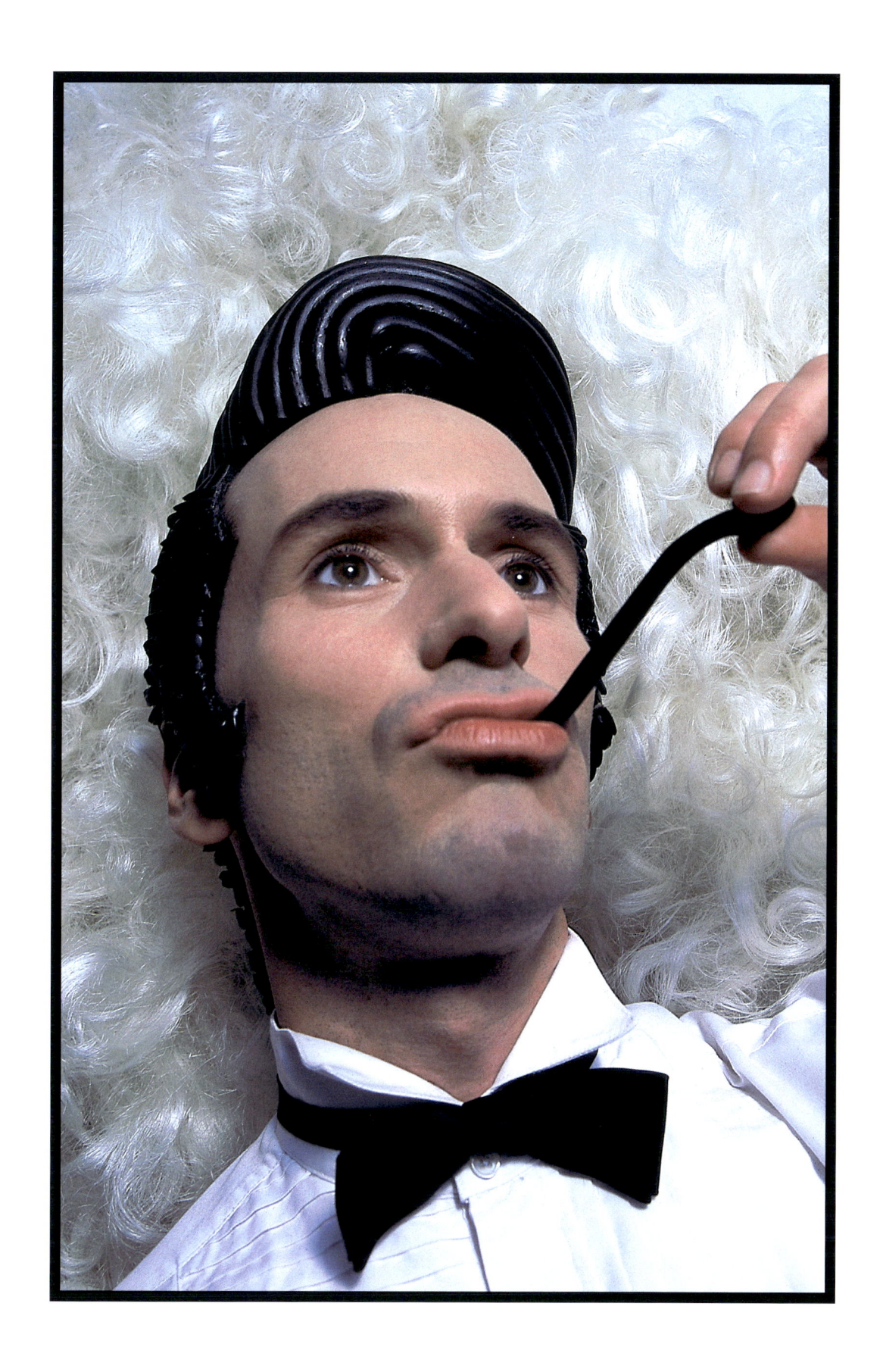

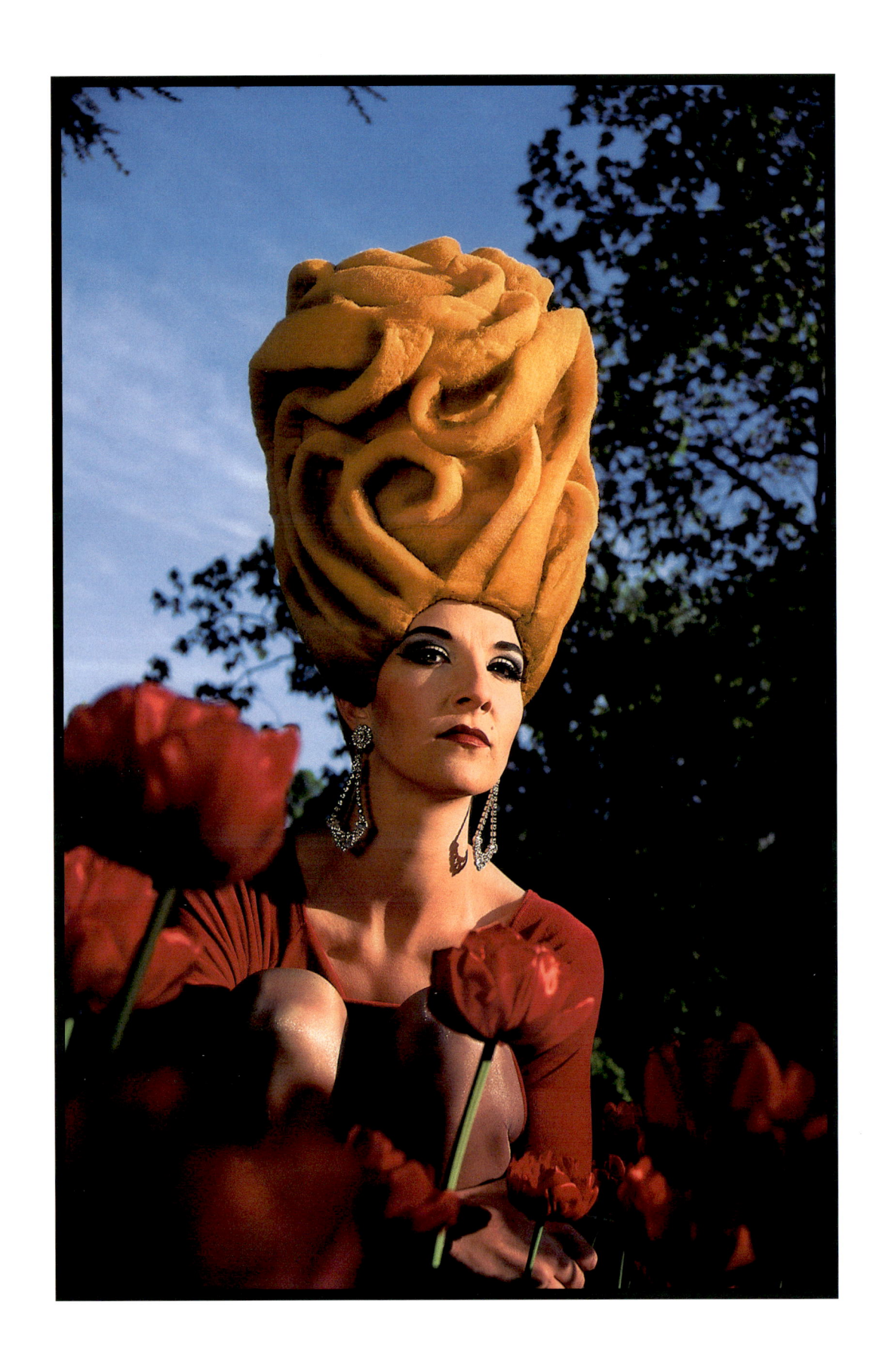

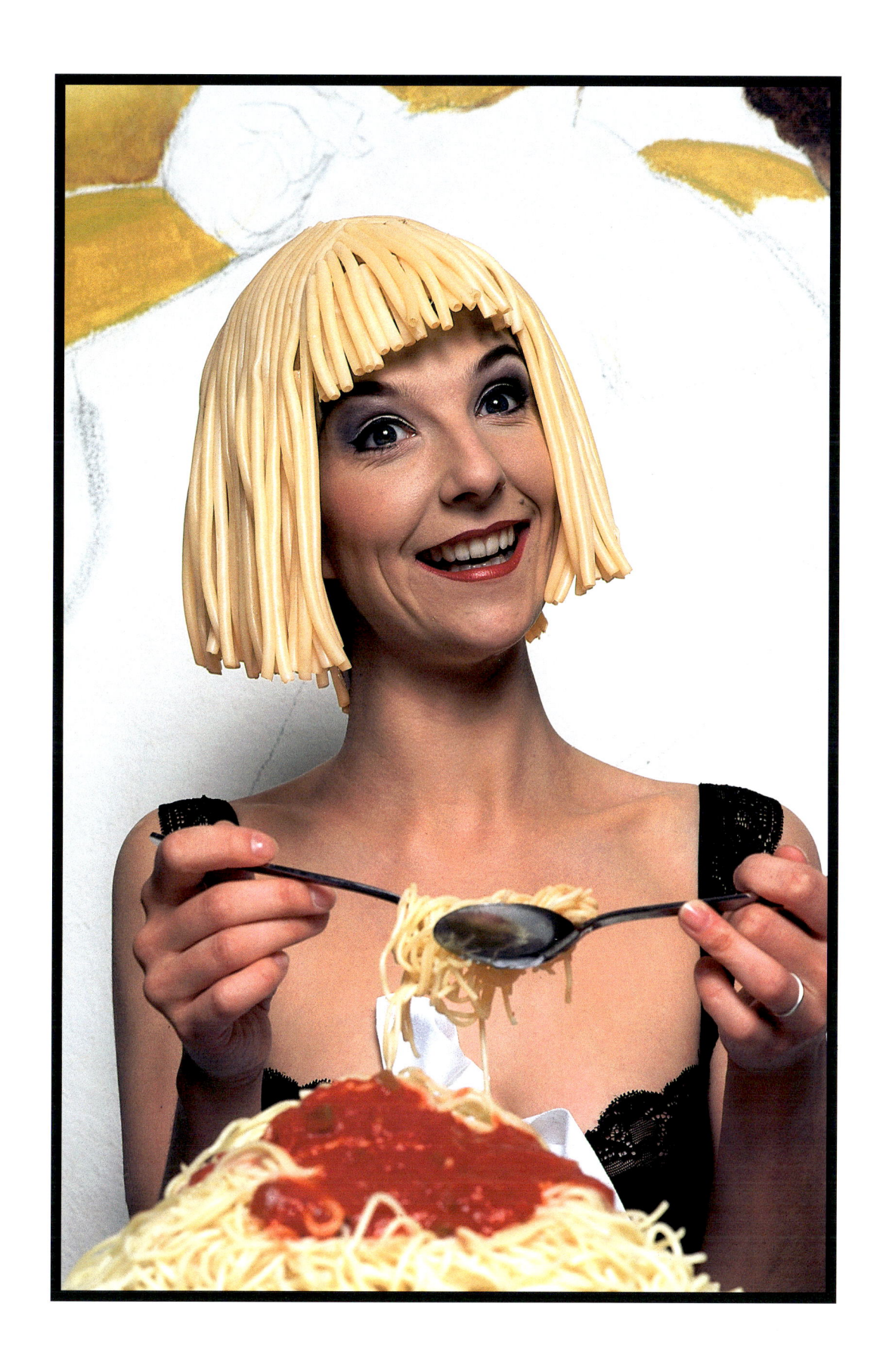

Hairy – Hairier – Hairiest

PEOPLE always want to have exactly what has not been given unto them. An entire guild lives as mediator between reality and wishful thinking. With their skills they try to make up for that which nature has so steadfastly withheld.

In the Goldwell lab which tests permanents, chemists check new tinctures for substance loss, stretching, and tearing. 80,000 strands of hair are necessary to test a hair color's durability. In 1909, the Frenchman, Eugène Schuller, developed the first hair color for the market. This was the matrix for the L'Oréal company. In the fifties, colored hair was considered wicked. Only 7% of American women colored their hair; today 75% change their hair color.

115

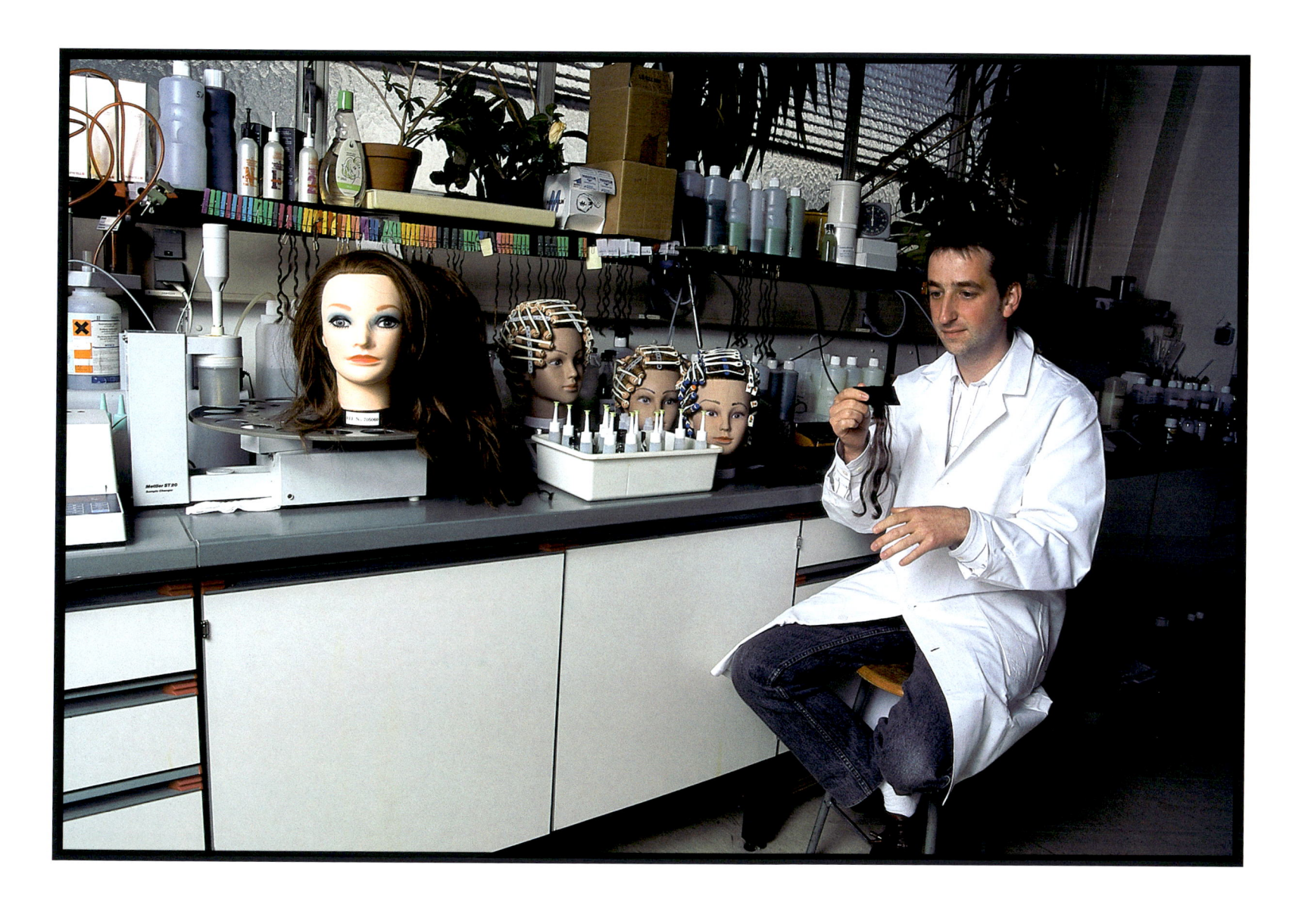

"AFRO SHOP" in the Adenauerallee in Hamburg has a flourishing hair-business: hair-care and styling products are for sale, as well as artificial and real hair. Even groceries and baby service are included.

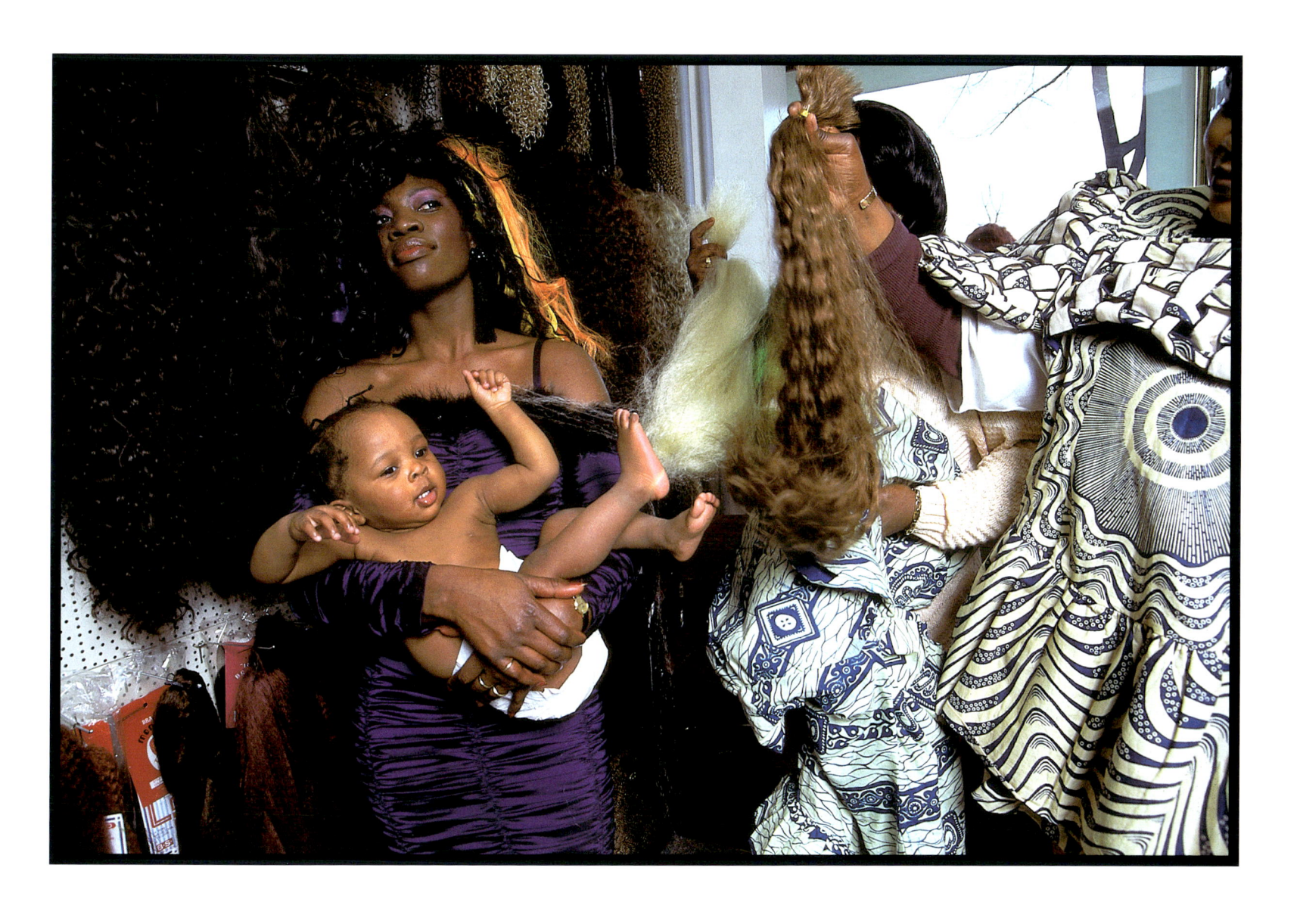

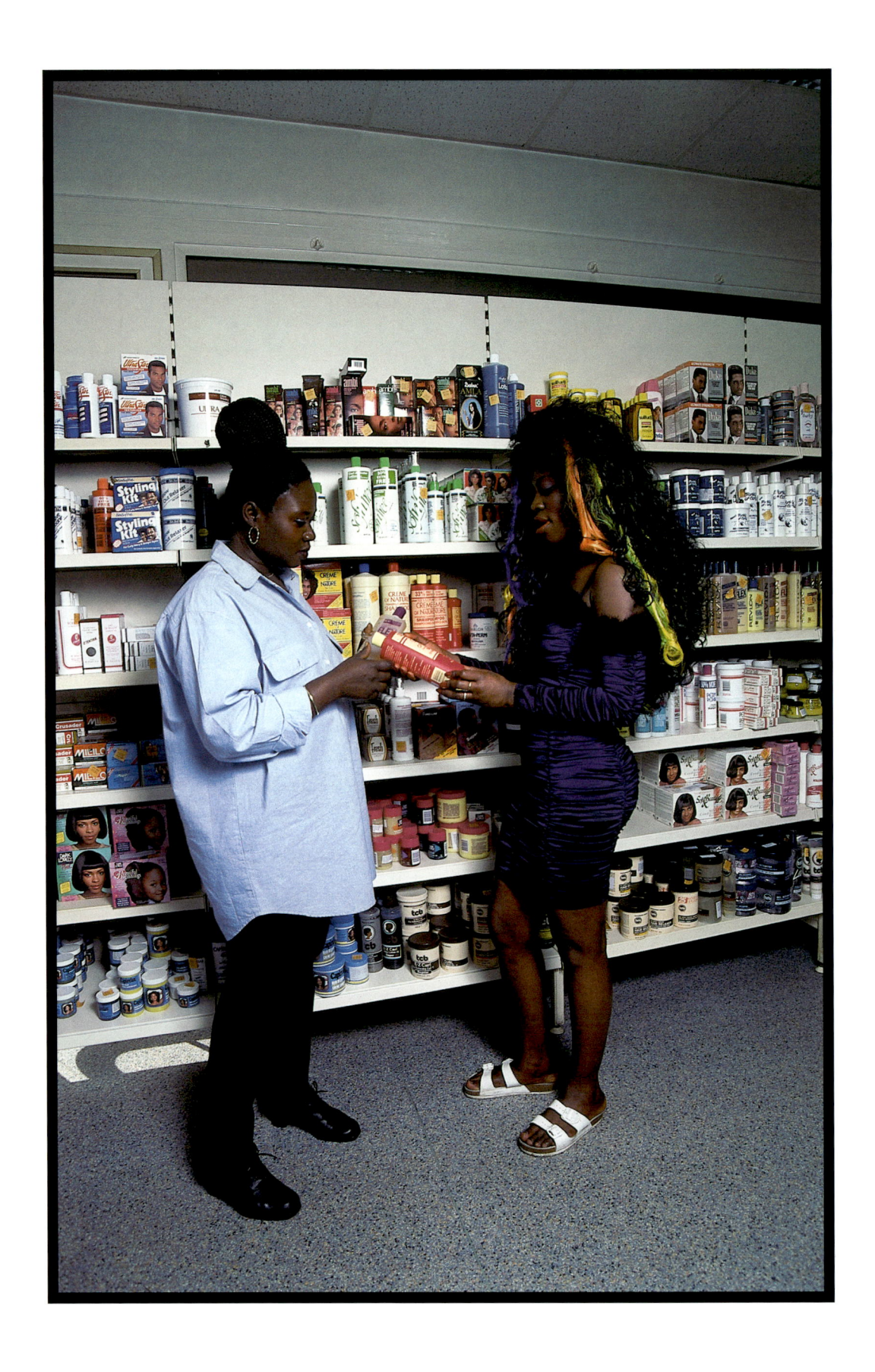

119

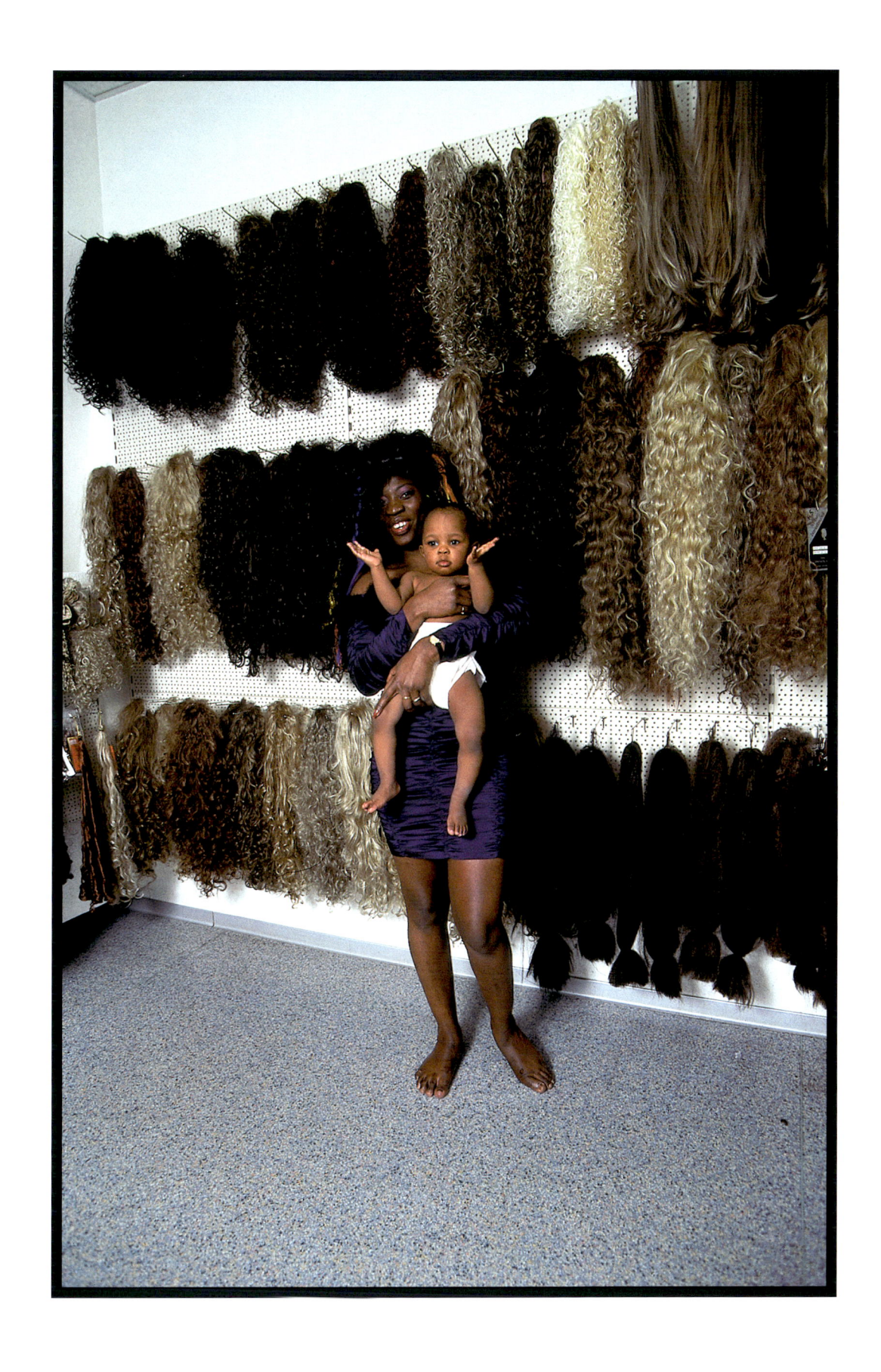

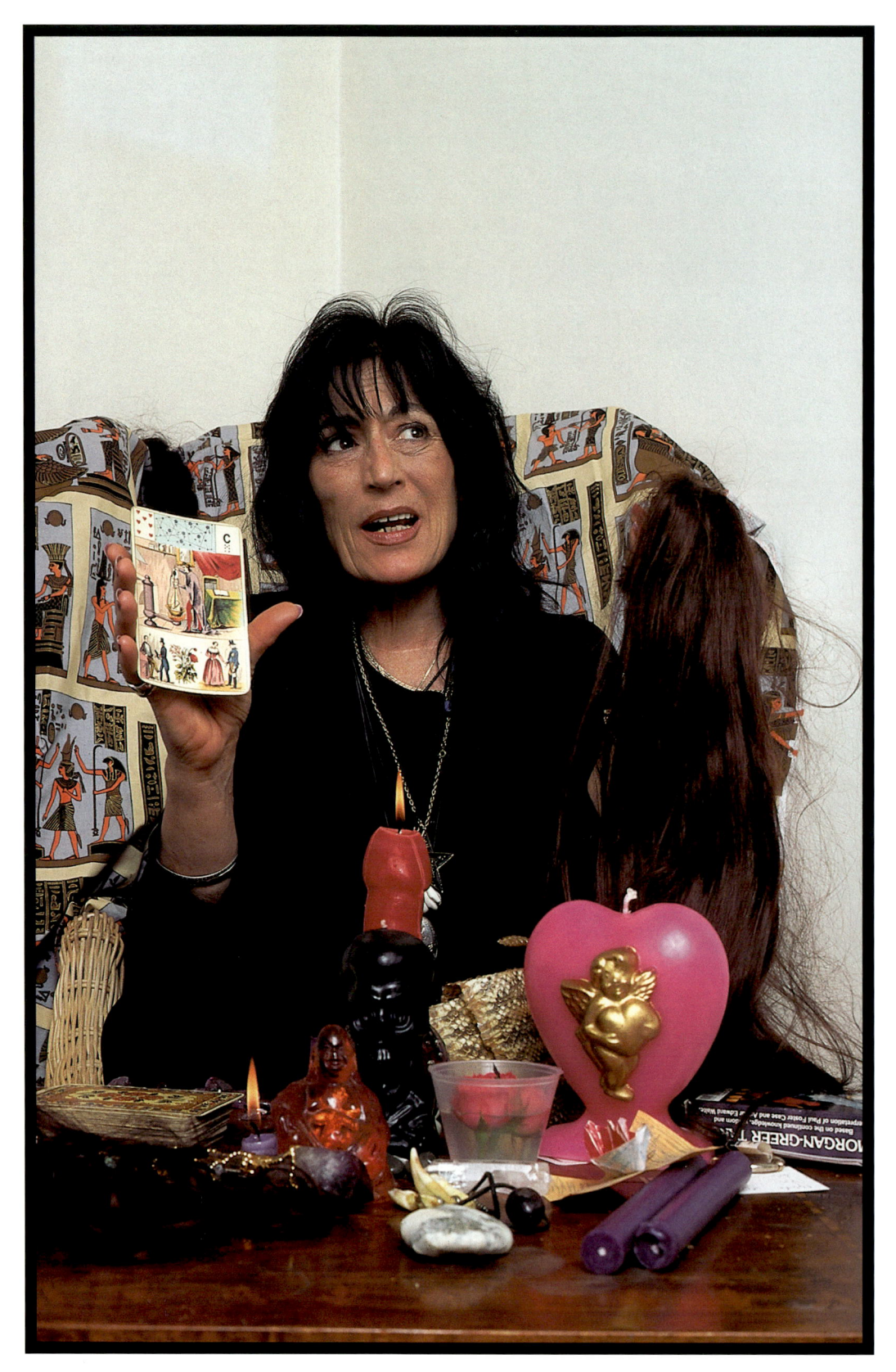

FOR SANDRA, who calls herself a witch, hair is a significant remedy in her world of magic. She tries to cure broken hearts in various rituals with the hairs of her customers' partners. The magician from Munich believes in hair-power so much that she would never leave one behind in her hair-brush. Far too great is her fear that someone might harm her or gain power over her.

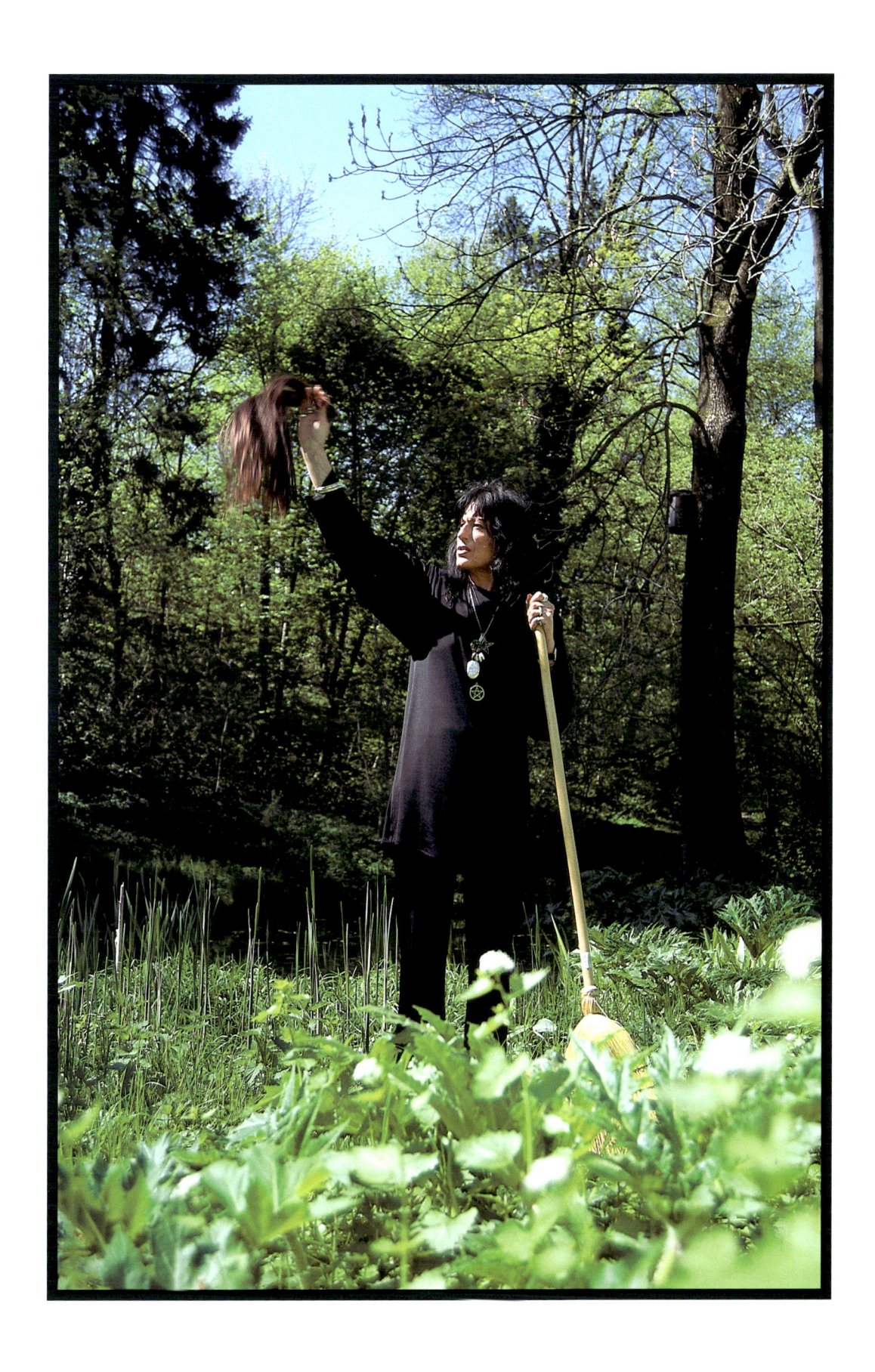

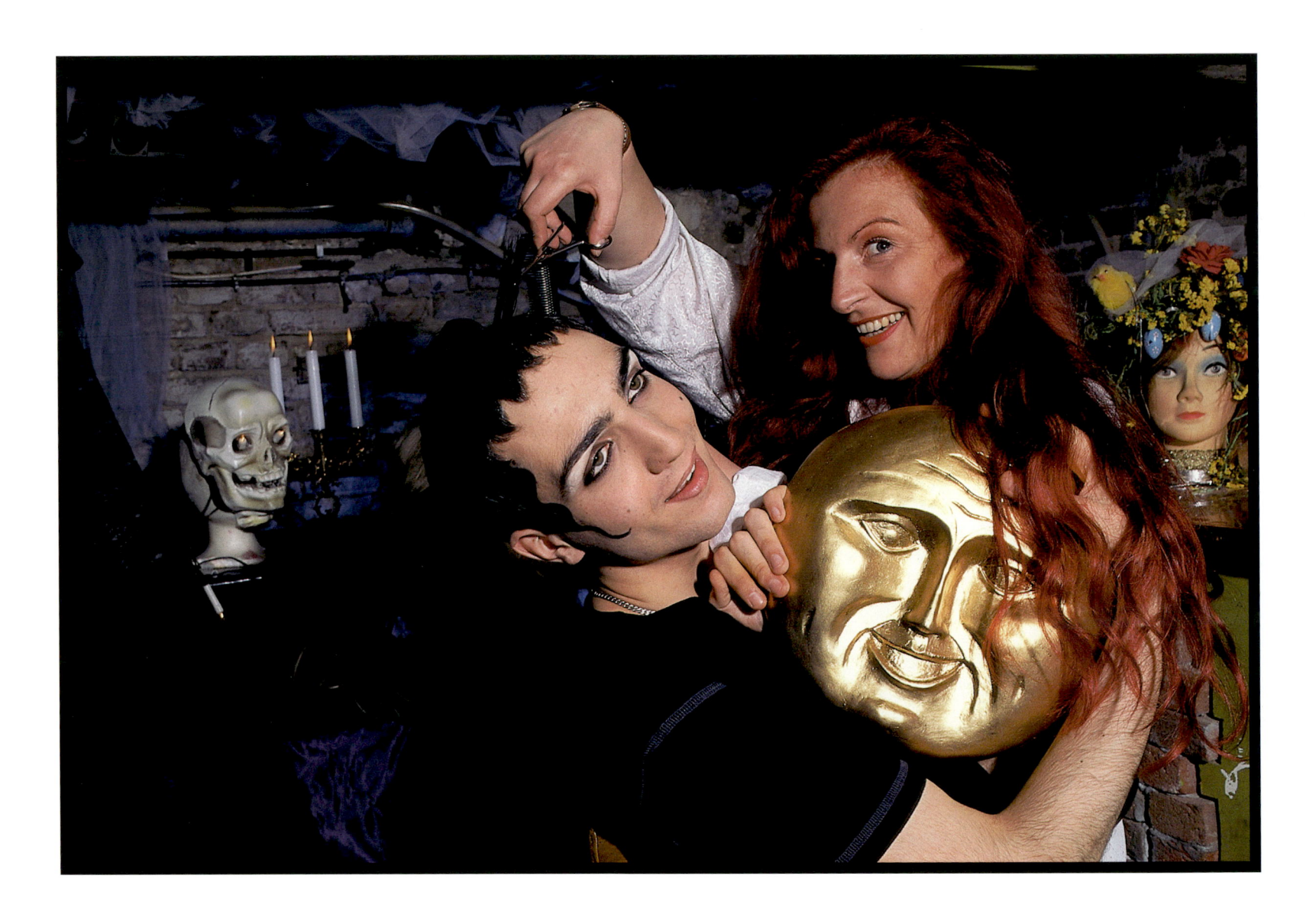

UTE JACOBS from Berlin swears by the magical power of the full moon. On such nights, she organizes occult haircutting sessions with oracles and love potions.

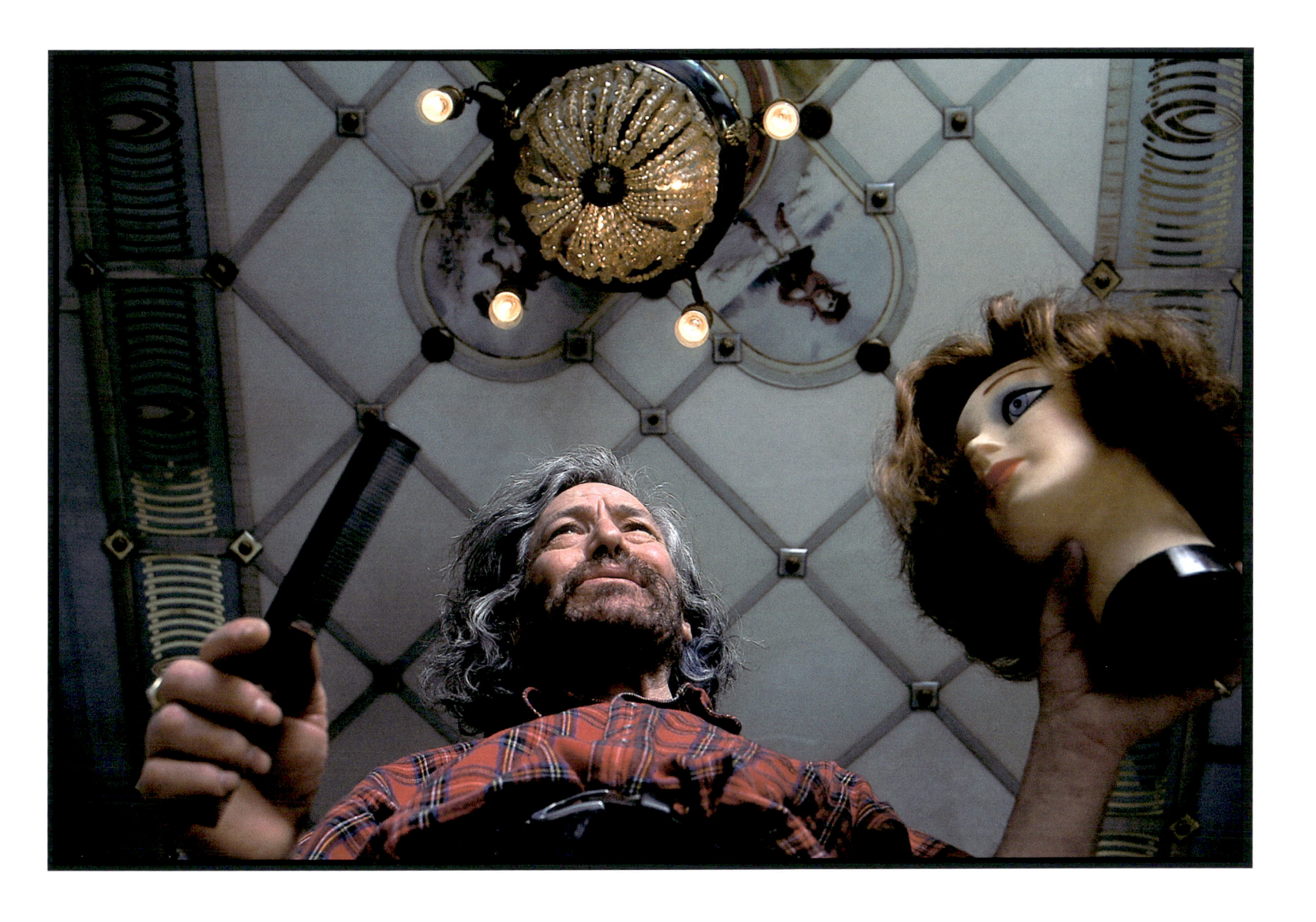

THE GREEK hairdresser and wig-maker from "Zobo," located in Eppendorfer Weg in Hamburg considers himself a philosopher. His relationship to artificial hair is totally relaxed. Unlike fellow countryman and theologian, Tertullian. In the second century A.D. he preached that all wigs served deception and were the devil's work.

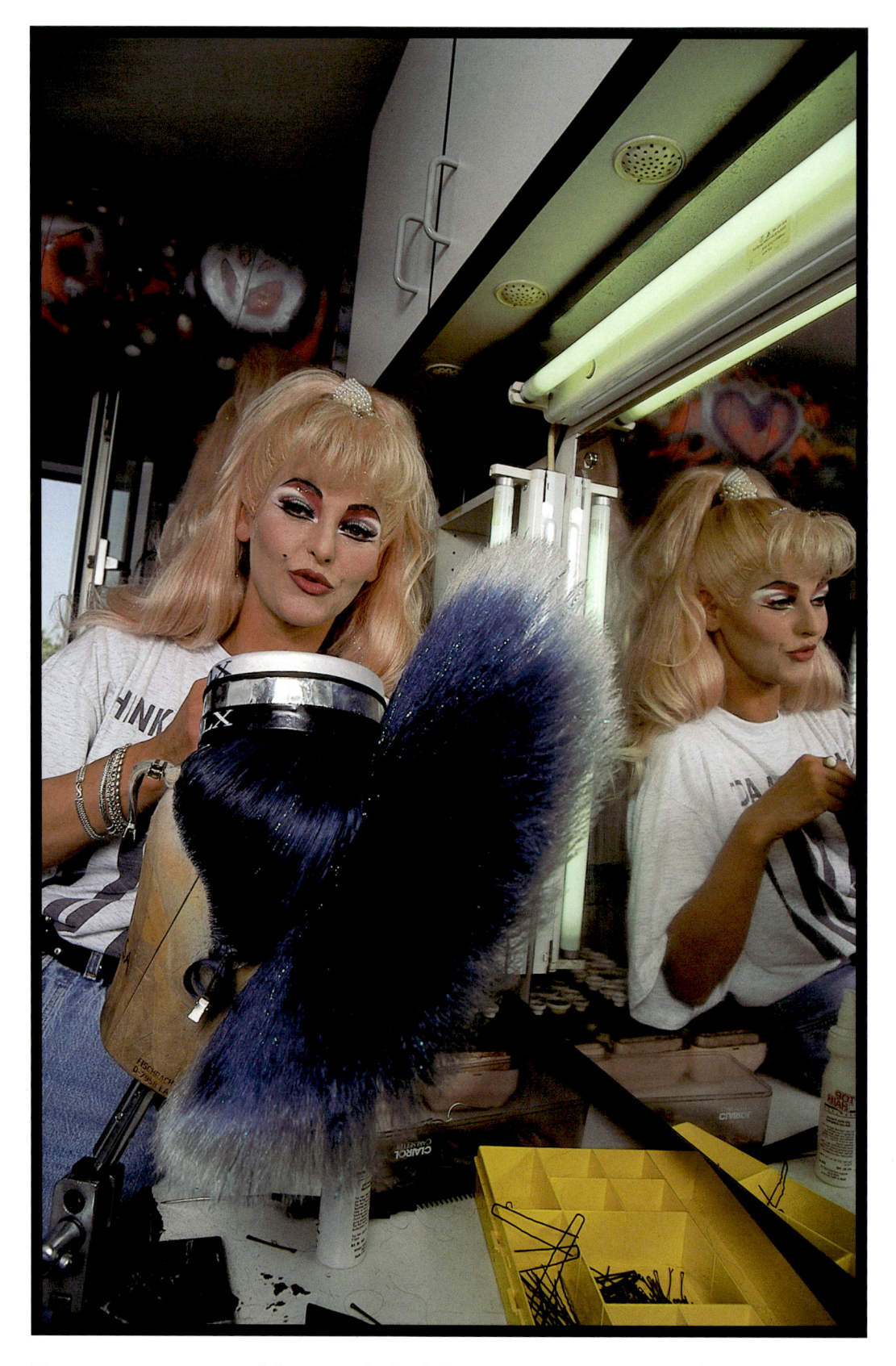

THE MAKE-UP artist of the musical "Starlight Express," running in Bochum, is quite busy. For the Locomotive World Championship he has to put on and secure all kinds of fantasy wigs made of buffalo and human hair. Then, after each show, he has to wash, dry, and re-style them all.

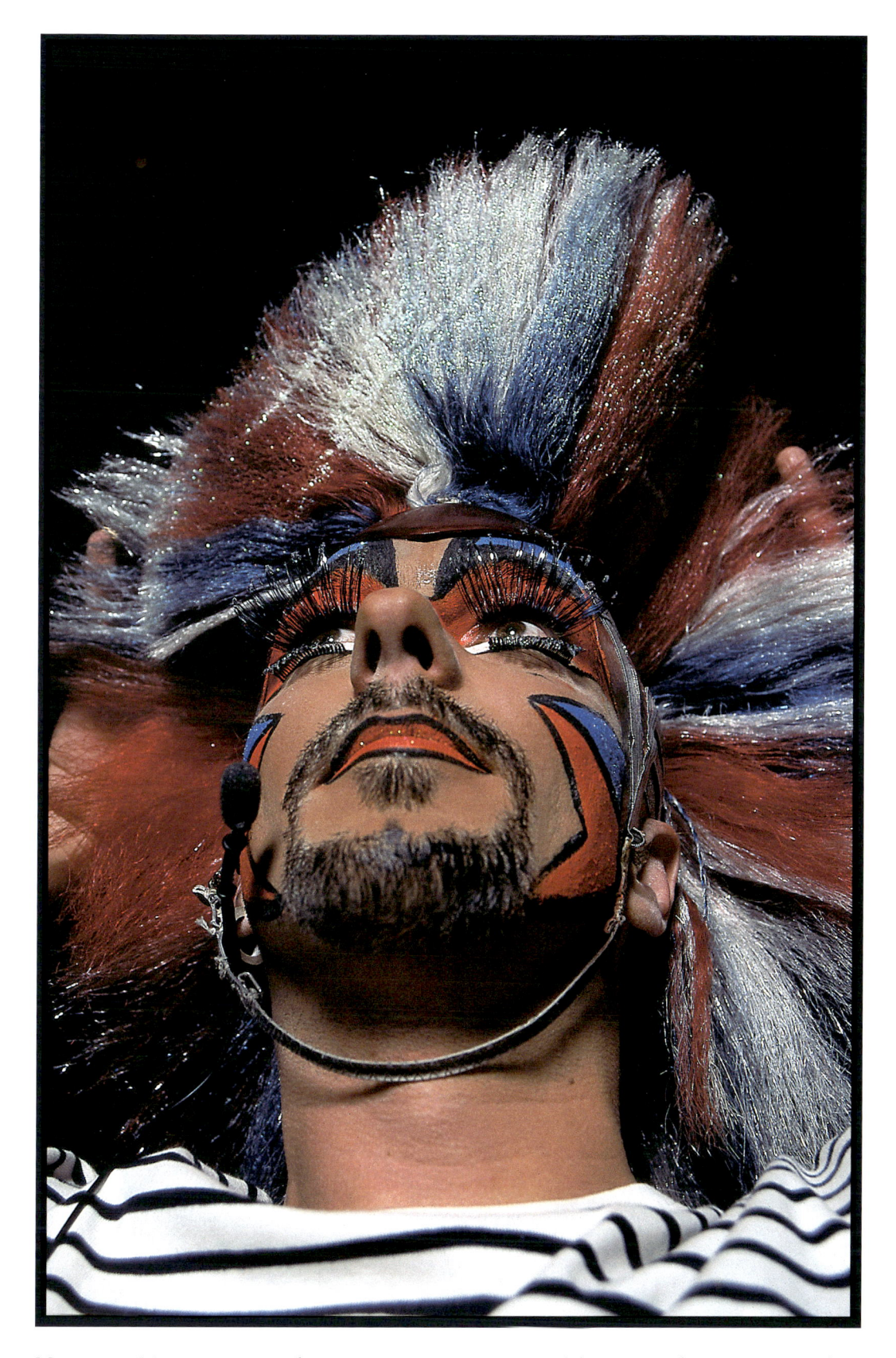

MARTIN MANNECK, Make-Up Director, presents "Elektra's" outfit, a super modern electric locomotive. His assistant, Mickie, is responsible for the wig "Dinah," which depicts the dining car.

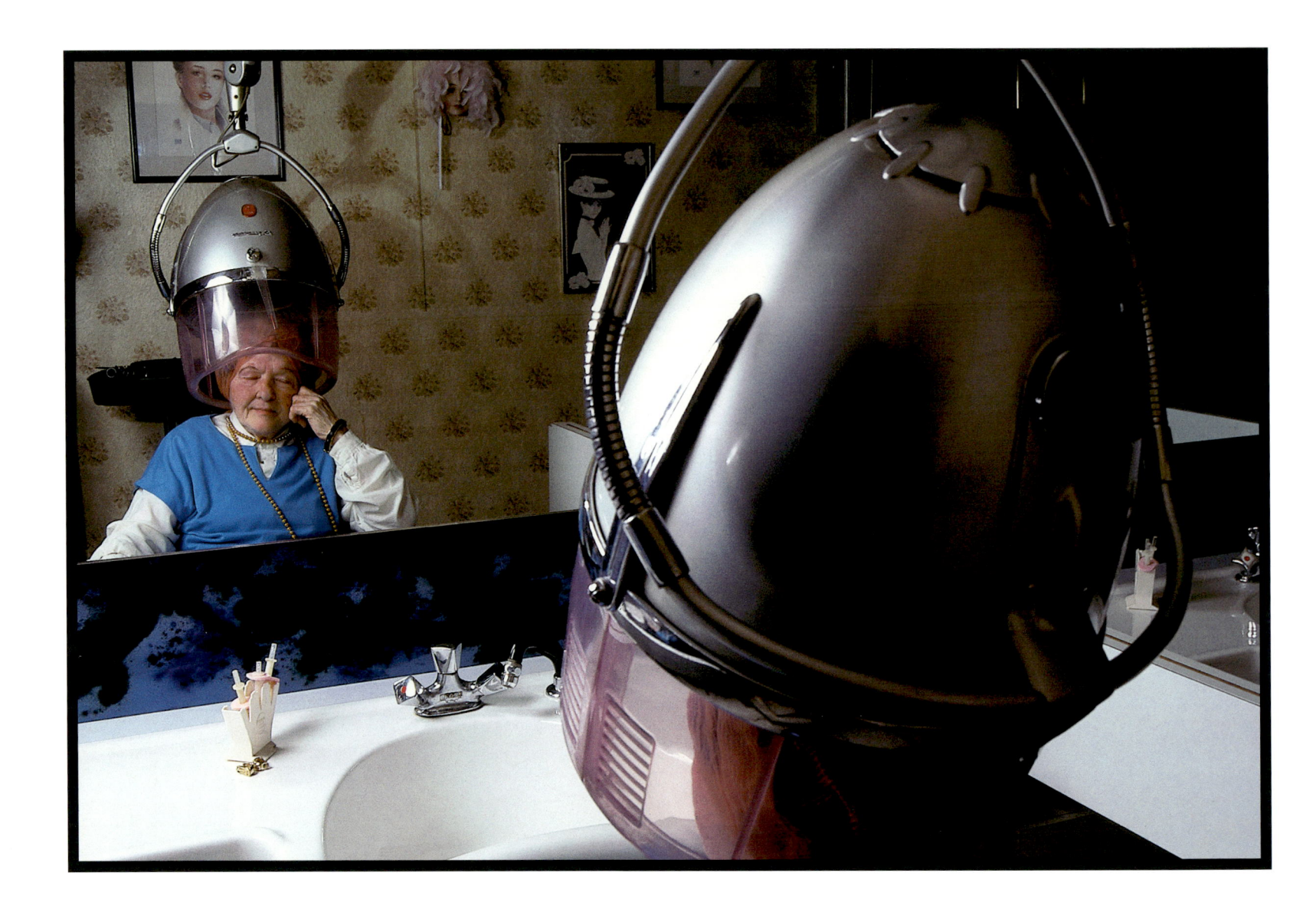

UNDER THE HOOD: totally absorbed in thought or taking a nap, young or old: the ladies all are waiting for the one and only: their permanent.

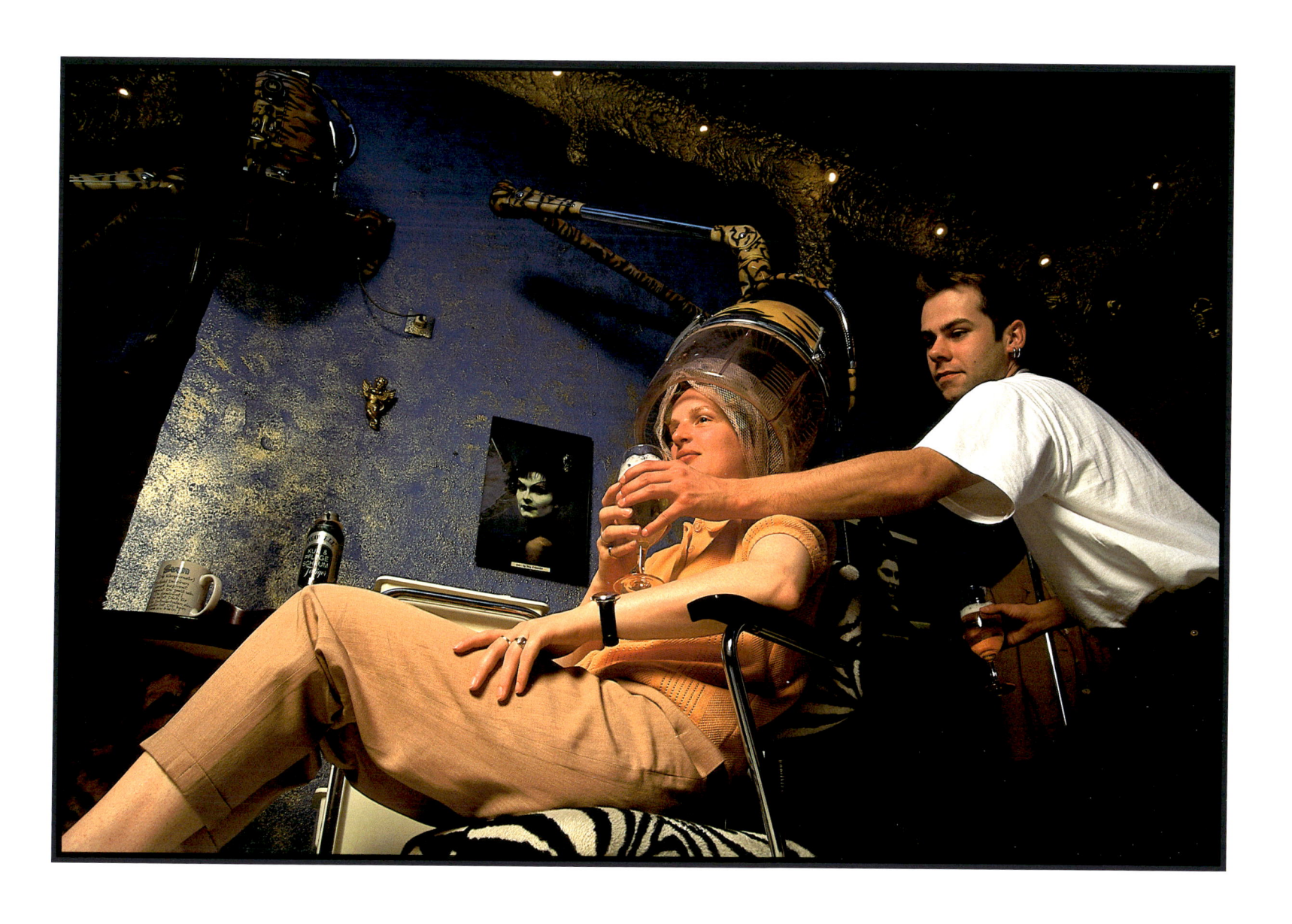

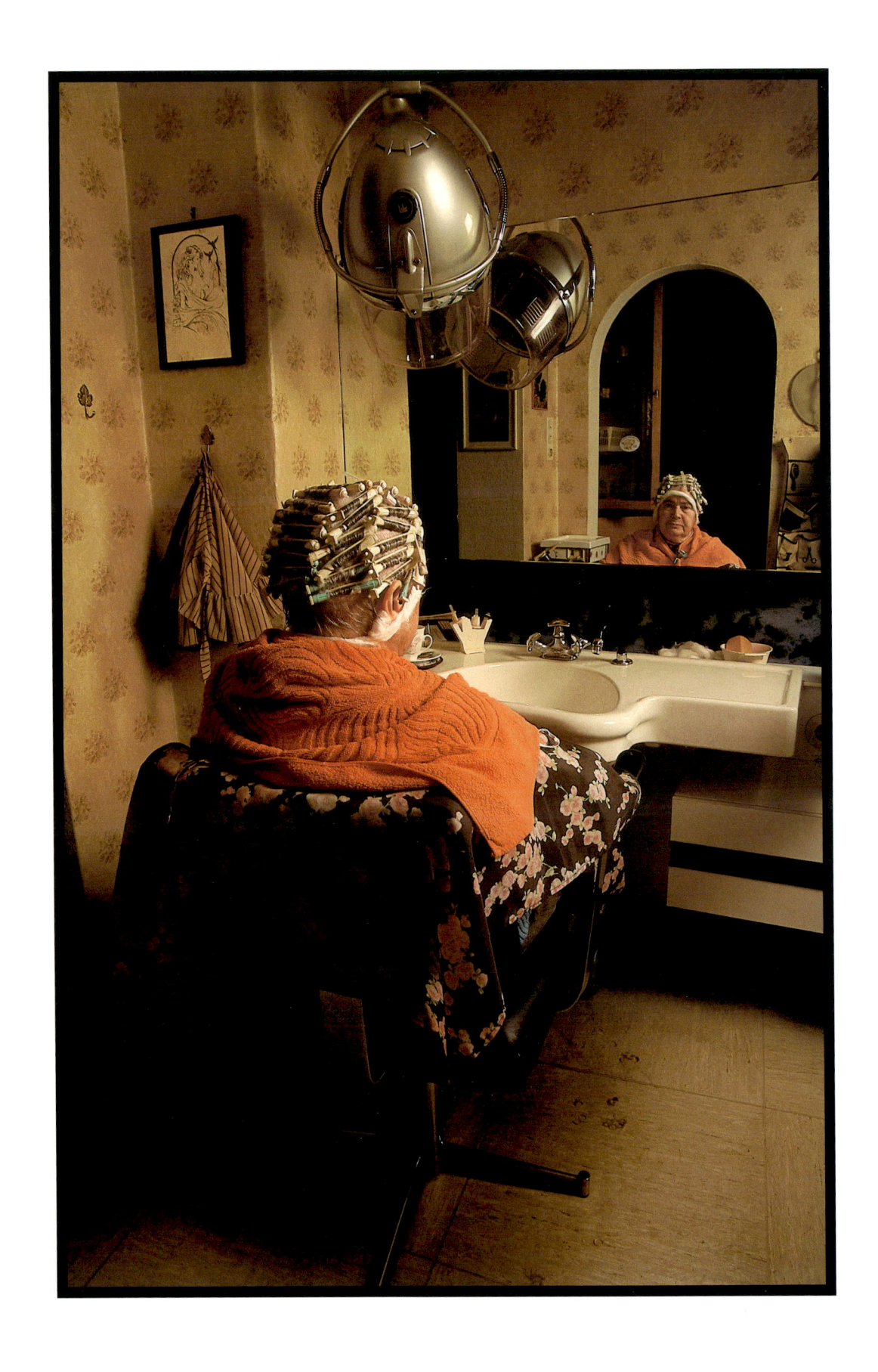

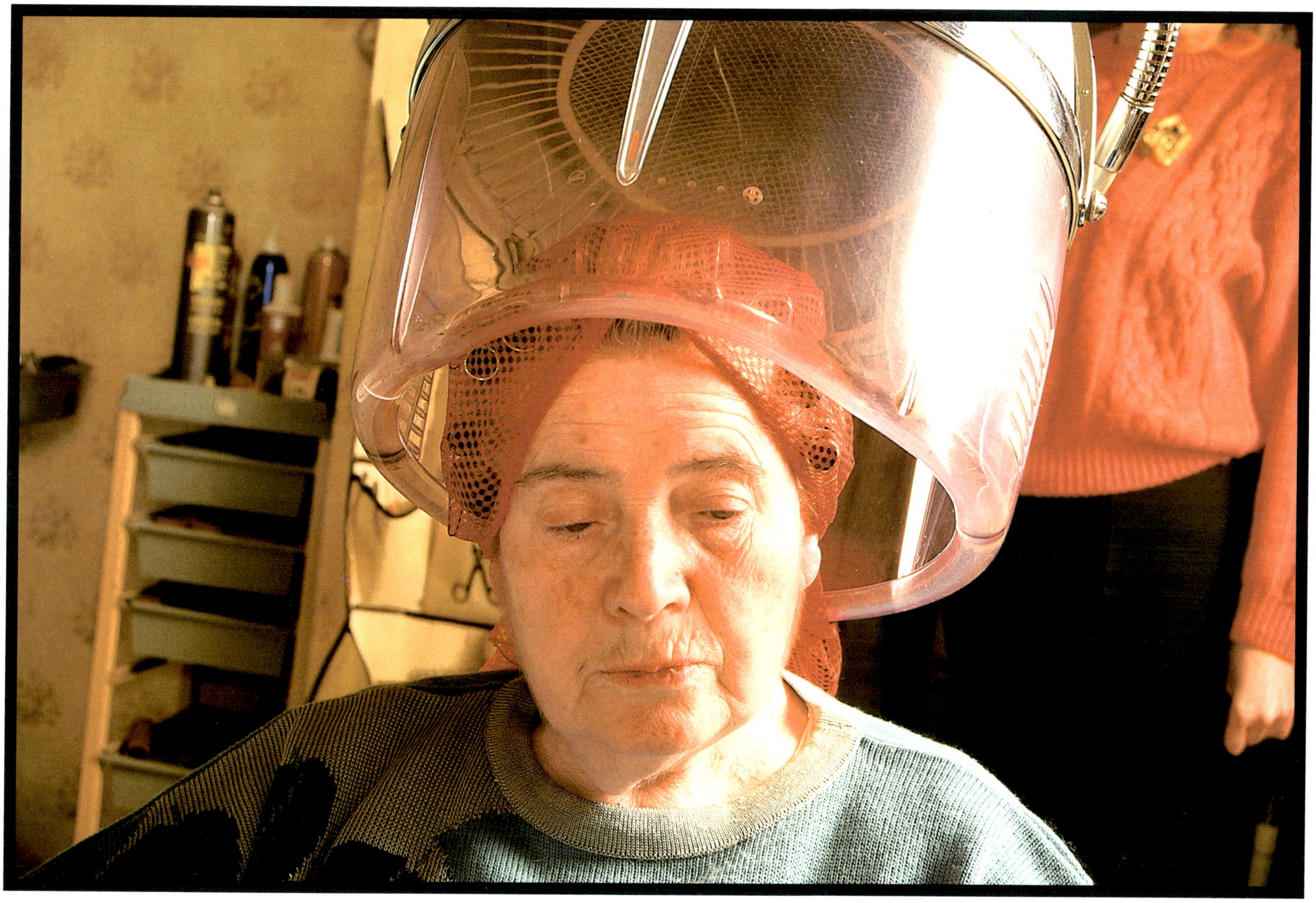

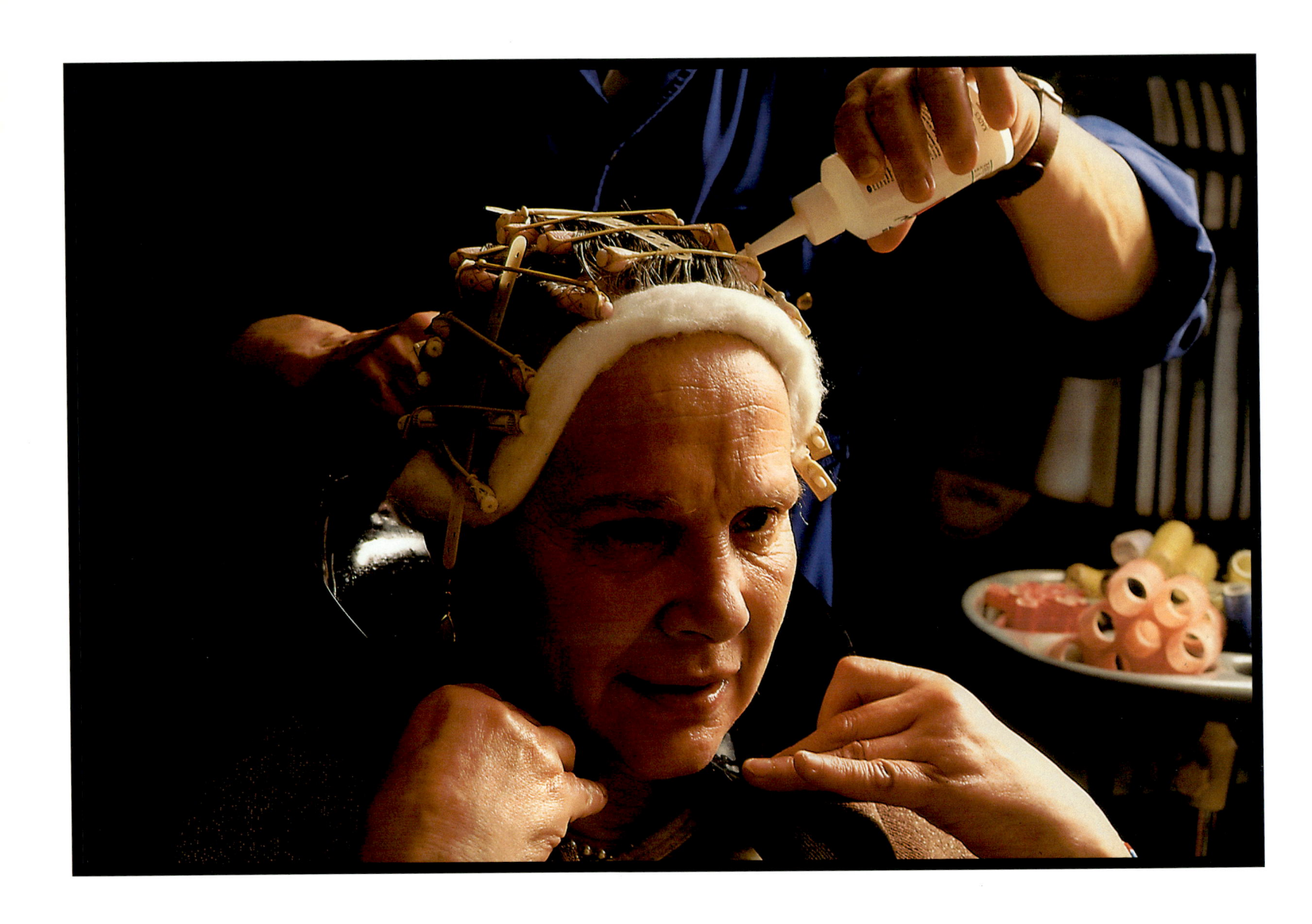

KRIBBELKRÄUSCHEN "tickly curls" are a favorite hairstyle of elderly women, who put up with hours of treatment with caustic, horrible-smelling tinctures to get them.

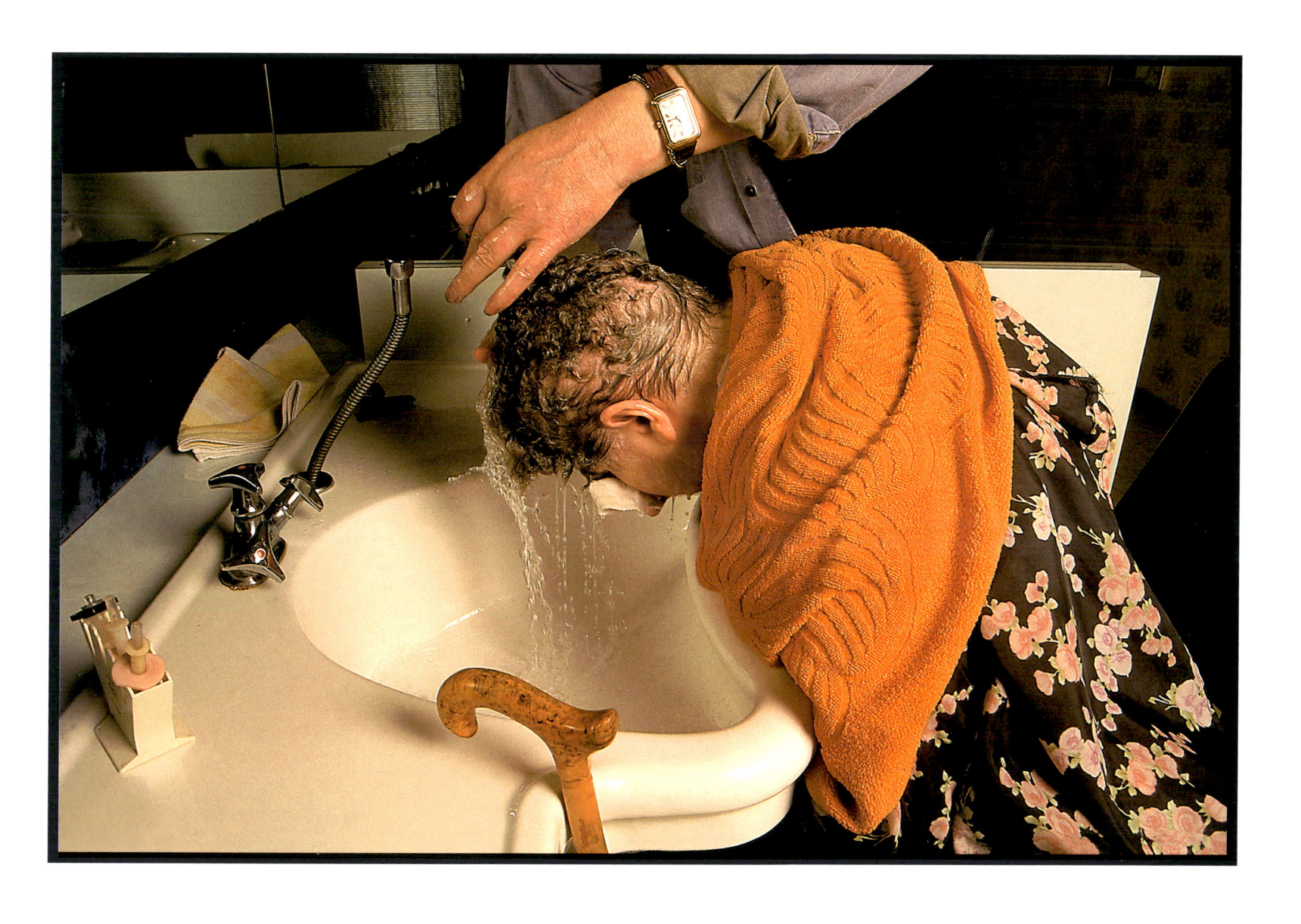

"A KISS WITHOUT A BEARD IS LIKE SOUP WITHOUT SALT," is the motto of the First Höfener Bart- und Schnorresclub e. V. 1985. And to ensure that women get the message, the members of this largest beard-and-moustache club in the world brush, trim and treat their facial hair with wax and mink-oil daily. Mirror, mirror on the wall, who has the handsomest beard of all?

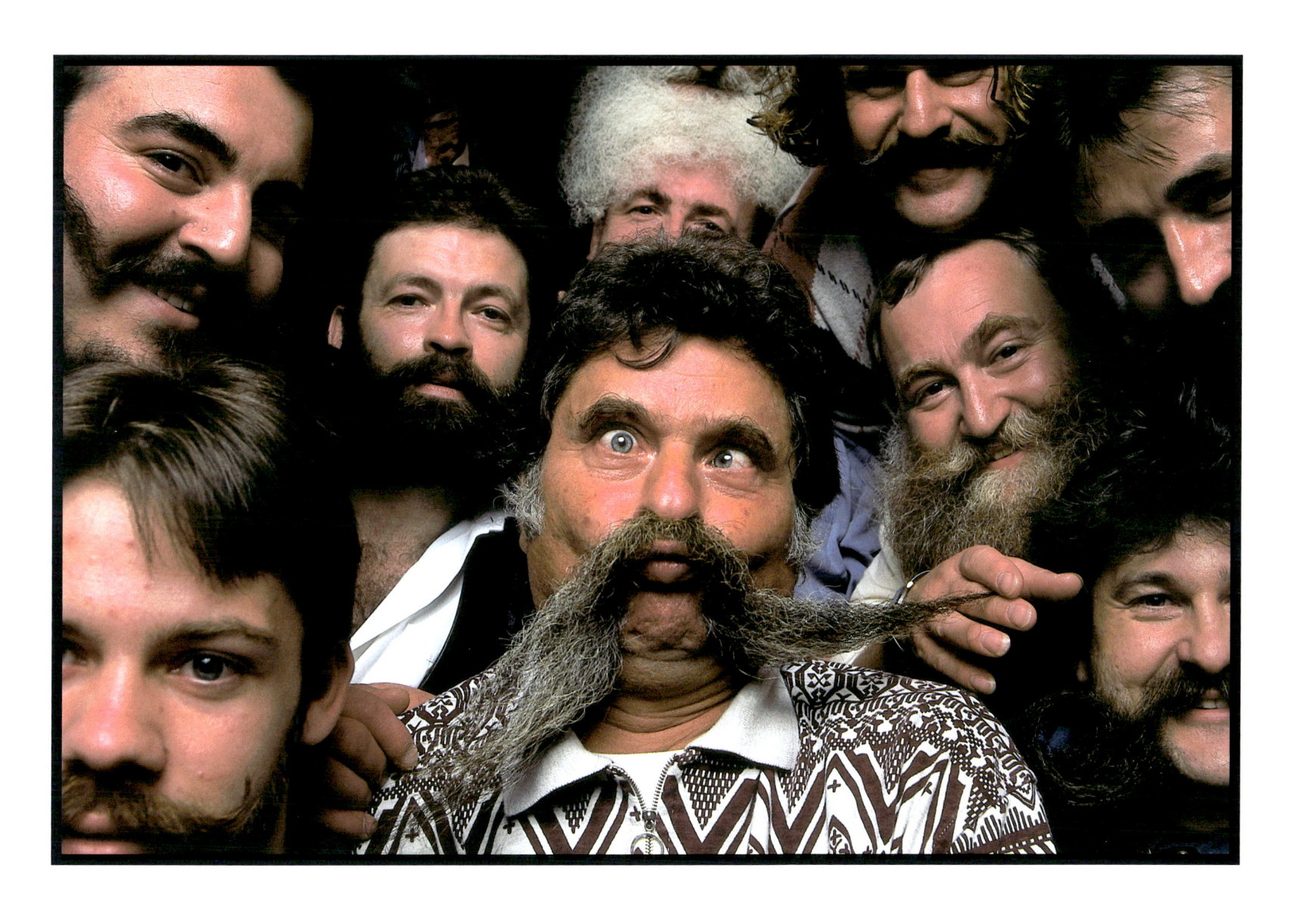

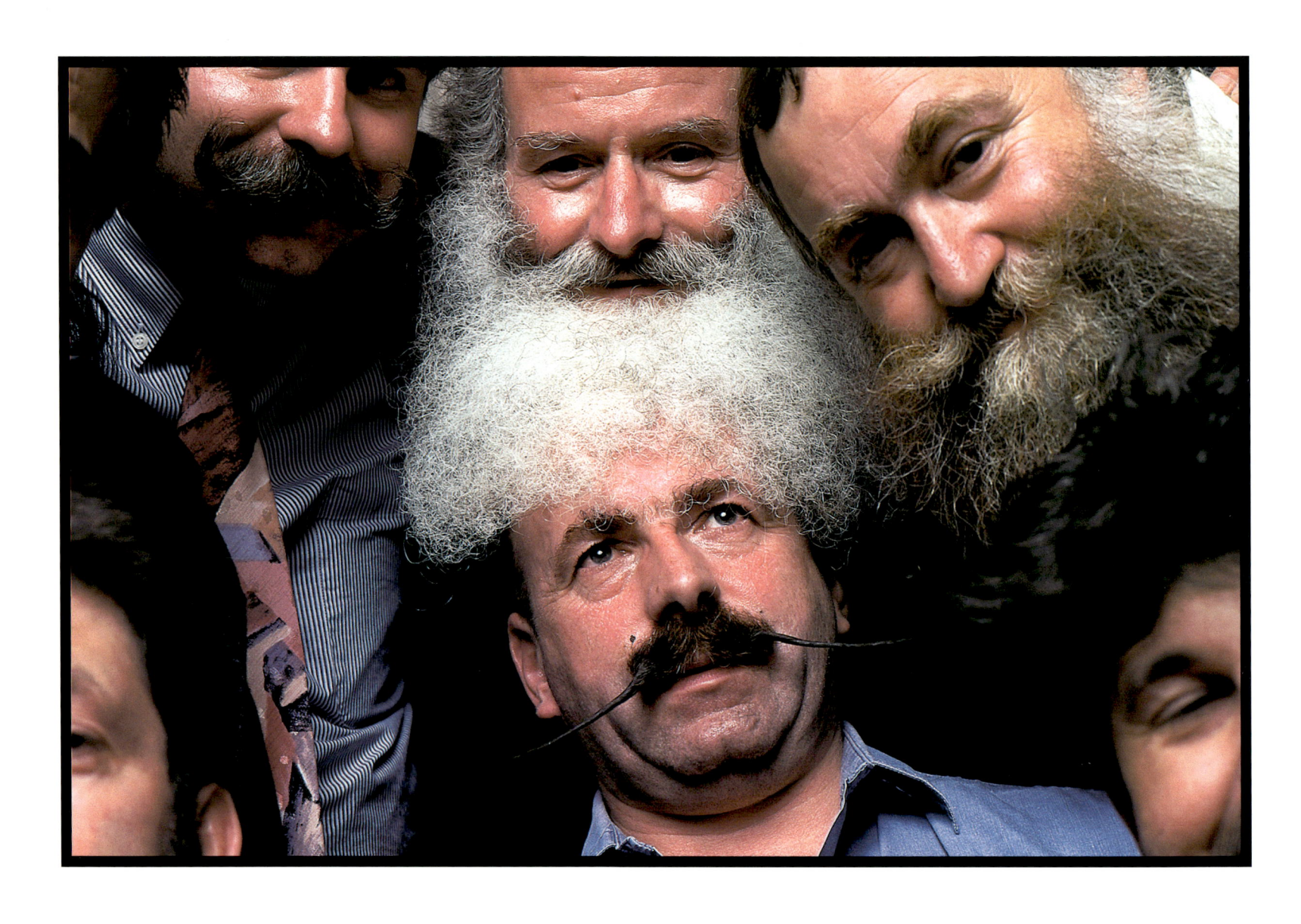

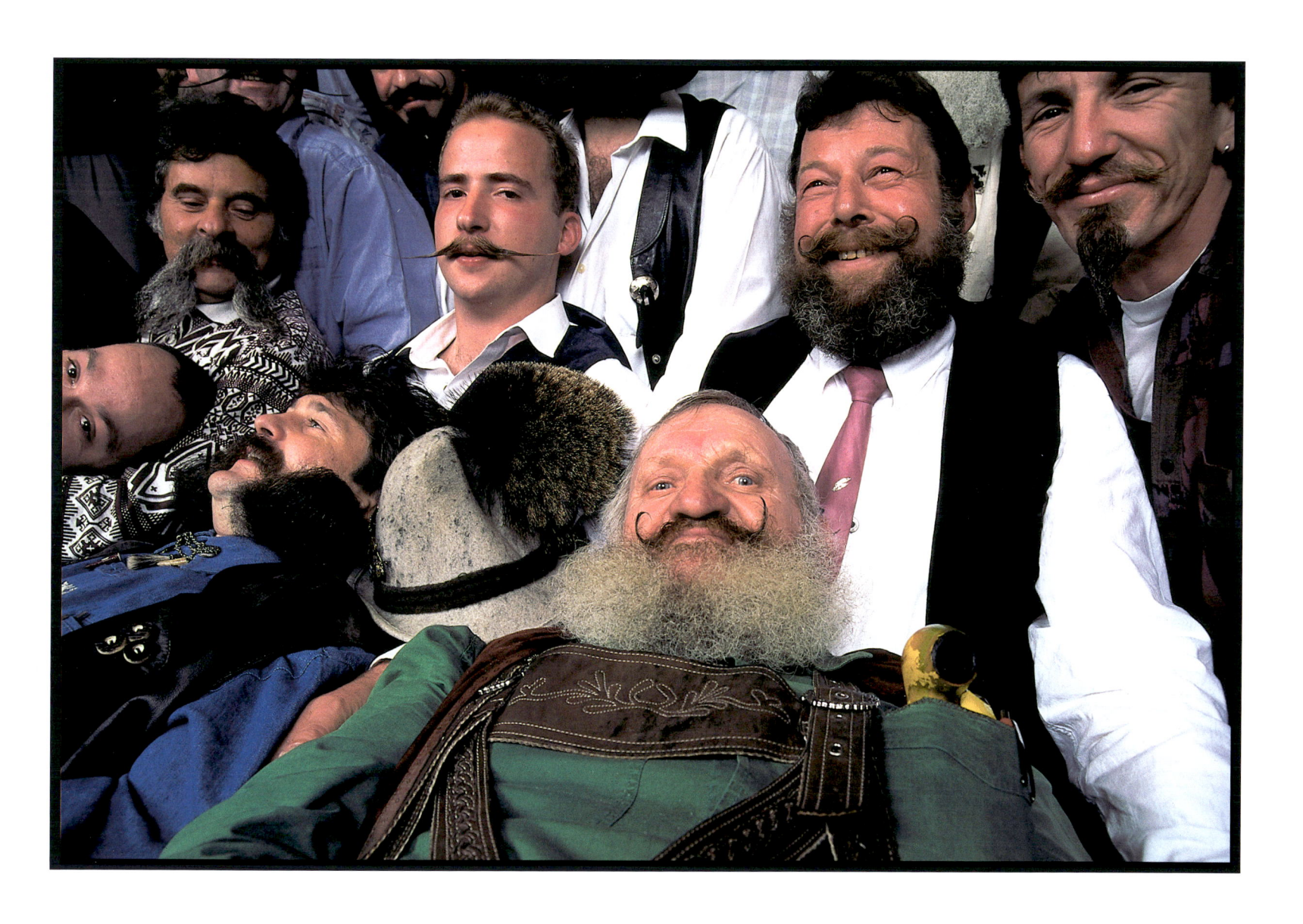

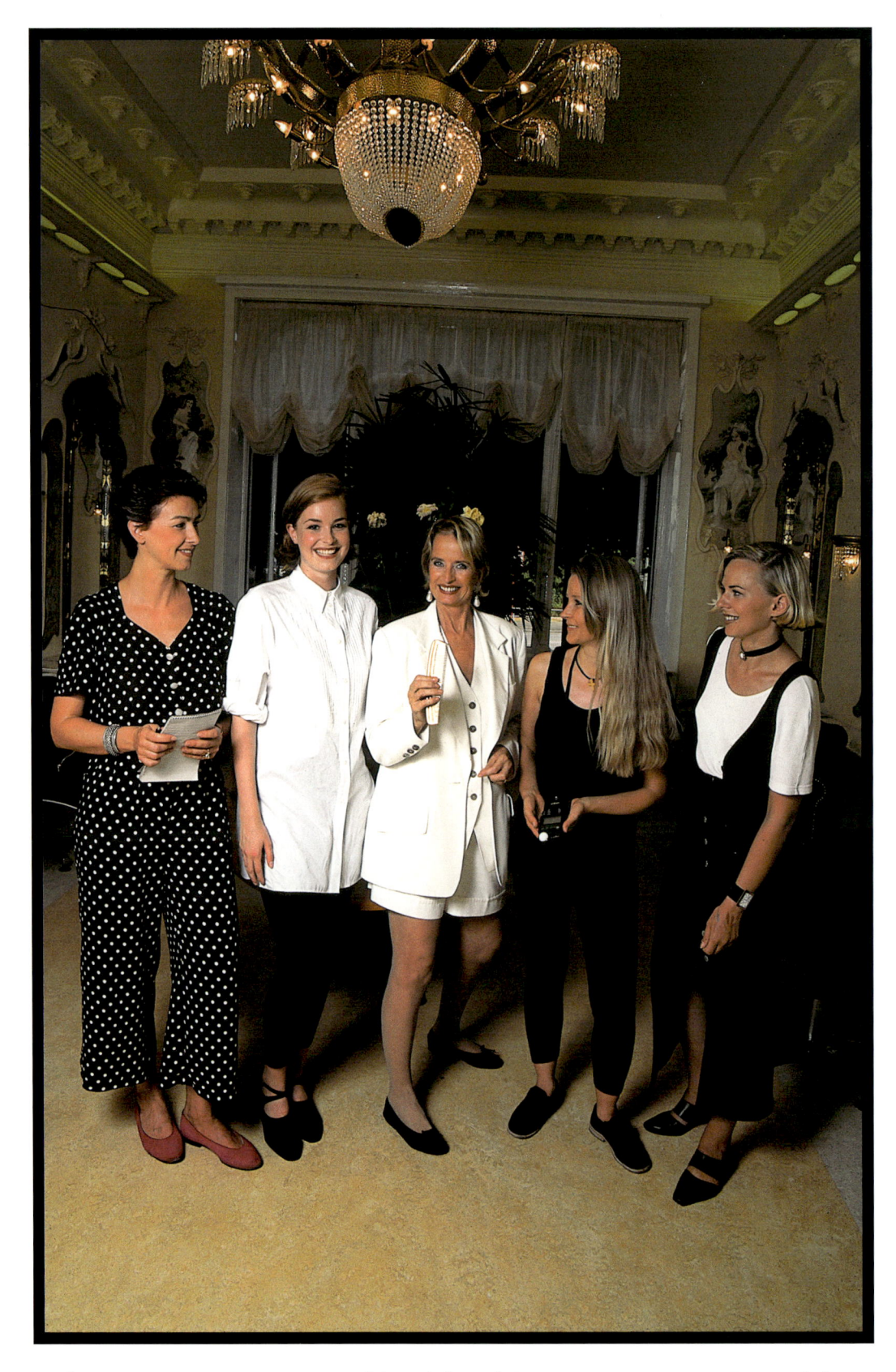

Authors BEATE BROSCHE, second from left, and GUDRUN PATRICIA POTT, left, with hairstylist Marlies Möller and stylists at the MM Salon in Hamburg.

BEATE BROSCHE

Born in 1964, studies in Visual Communications at the Gesamthochschule Kassel (Prof. Floris M. Neusüss); further studies at the Hochschule für Bildende Künste Braunschweig; studies in Photography under Prof. Michael Ruetz; earned university diploma as a designer; has worked as a freelance photographer for magazines and advertising agencies since 1992; member of the "Focus" photo and press agency in Hamburg.

GUDRUN PATRICIA POTT

Born in 1959, studies in Medieval and Modern History and Political Science at the Universität Hamburg; worked during this period on documentation for the weekly magazine *Der Spiegel*; voluntary training at the *Hamburger Morgenpost* newspaper and training in journalism at the Akademie für Publizistik, Hamburg; an editor for *Stern* magazine for five years; has worked as a freelance journalist in Hamburg since 1995.

The authors received an award from the Art Directors' Club of Germany for a *Stern* feature on hairstyling salons in Germany.

ACKNOWLEDGMENT

Thanks are due to our publisher of choice Edition Stemmle for believing in our project. And especially to the Goldwell company whose enthusiastic support enabled us to publish this book.

Beate Brosche and Gudrun Patricia Pott

Copyright © 1998 by
EDITION STEMMLE AG, 8802 Kilchberg/Zurich, Switzerland

All rights reserved.
No part of this book may be reproduced or transmitted in any form or by any means, electronic or mechanical, including photocopy, recording or any other information storage and retrieval system, without the written permission of the publisher.

Reproduction copyright by Beate Brosche
Text copyright by Gudrun Patricia Pott
Translation from the German by Suzanne R. Goff
Art direction by Beate Brosche and Michael Grübeling, Hamburg, Germany
Photolithography by Pre Press Design AG, St. Gallen, Switzerland
Printed and bound by Kündig Druck AG, Baar, Switzerland
ISBN 3-908162-78-5